T0200397

Transitions of Care for Patients with Neurological Diagnoses

Editor

SONJA E. STUTZMAN

NURSING CLINICS
OF NORTH AMERICA

www.nursing.theclinics.com

Consulting Editor
STEPHEN D. KRAU

September 2019 • Volume 54 • Number 3

ELSEVIER

1600 John F. Kennedy Boulevard • Suite 1800 • Philadelphia, Pennsylvania, 19103-2899

http://www.theclinics.com

NURSING CLINICS OF NORTH AMERICA Volume 54, Number 3
September 2019 ISSN 0029-6465, ISBN-13: 978-0-323-67898-8

Editor: Kerry Holland
Developmental Editor: Casey Potter

Nursing Clinics of North America (ISSN 0029-6465) is published quarterly by Elsevier Inc., 360 Park Avenue South, New York, NY 10010-1710. Months of issue are March, June, September, and December. Periodicals postage paid at New York, NY and additional mailing offices. Subscription price per year is, $163.00 (US individuals), $491.00 (US institutions), $275.00 (international individuals), $598.00 (international institutions), $231.00 (Canadian individuals), $598.00 (Canadian institutions), $100.00 (US students), and $135.00 (international students). To receive student/resident rate, orders must be accompanied by name of affiliated institution, date of term, and the signature of program/residency coordinator on institution letterhead. Orders will be billed at individual rate until proof of status is received. Foreign air speed delivery is included in all *Clinics* subscription prices. All prices are subject to change without notice. **POSTMASTER:** Send address changes to *Nursing Clinics*, Elsevier Health Sciences Division, Subscription Customer Service, 3251 Riverport Lane, Maryland Heights, MO 63043. **Customer Service: Telephone: 1-800-654-2452** (U.S. and Canada); **1-314-447-8871 (outside U.S. and Canada). Fax: 1-314-447-8029. E-mail: journalscustomerservice-usa@elsevier.com** (for print support) and **journalsonlinesupport-usa@elsevier.com** (for online support).

Nursing Clinics of North America is covered in *EMBASE/Excerpta Medica, MEDLINE/PubMed (Index Medicus), Social Sciences Citation Index, Current Contents, ASCA, Cumulative Index to Nursing, RNdex Top 100,* and Allied Health Literature and International Nursing Index (INI).

Contributors

CONSULTING EDITOR

STEPHEN D. KRAU, PhD, RN, CNE
Associate Professor (Ret), Vanderbilt University School of Nursing, Nashville, Tennessee, USA

EDITOR

SONJA E. STUTZMAN, PhD
Clinical Research Manager, O'Donnell Brain Institute, The University of Texas Southwestern Medical Center, Dallas, Texas, USA

AUTHORS

MAIGHDLIN W. ANDERSON, DNP, ACNP-BC
University of Pittsburgh School of Nursing, Pittsburgh, Pennsylvania, USA

JUANA BORJA-GONZALEZ, RN, MSN, PhD(c)
Instructor Professor, Nursing Department, Universidad del Norte, Barranquilla, Colombia

KELLIE BRENDLE, RN, MS, CNS
Trauma/Critical Care Clinical Nurse Specialist, Stroke Clinical Nurse Specialist, Heart and Vascular Services, UC Davis Health, Sacramento, California, USA

MEGAN A. BRISSIE, DNP, RN, ACNP-BC, CEN
Acute Care Nurse Practitioner, Department of Neurosurgery, Duke University Health System, Duke Regional Hospital, Durham, North Carolina, USA

ROXANA DE LAS SALAS, RN, MSc, PhD(c)
Assistant Professor, Nursing Department, Universidad del Norte, Barranquilla, Colombia

ANITA FETZICK, RN, MSN, CCNS
Department of Neurological Surgery, Nurse Coordinator, Neurotrauma Clinical Trials Center, University of Pittsburgh, Pittsburgh, Pennsylvania, USA

NNEKA L. IFEJIKA, MD, MPH
Section Chief of Stroke Rehabilitation, Associate Professor, Physical Medicine and Rehabilitation, Neurology and Neurotherapeutics, Population and Data Sciences, The University of Texas Southwestern Medical Center, Dallas, Texas, USA

SHANNON B. JUENGST, PhD, CRC
Assistant Professor, Physical Medicine and Rehabilitation, The University of Texas Southwestern Medical Center, Dallas, Texas, USA

LORI KENNEDY MADDEN, PhD, RN, ACNP-BC, CCRN-K, CNRN
Clinical Nurse Scientist, Director, Center for Nursing Science, UC Davis Health,
Sacramento, California, USA

NORMA D. McNAIR, PhD, RN, ACNS-BC, FAHA
Former Clinical Nurse Specialist, Ronald Reagan UCLA Medical Center, Los Angeles,
California, USA

DIANE McLAUGHLIN, DNP, APRN-CNP, AGACNP-BC
Acute Care Nurse Practitioner, Neurocritical Care and Neurosurgery, The MetroHealth
System, Associate Clinical Professor, Case Western Reserve University, MetroHealth
Medical Center, Cleveland, Ohio, USA

MOLLY McNETT, PhD, RN, CNRN, FNCS
Professor, Clinical Nursing, Assistant Director, Implementation Science Core, The Helene
Fuld Health Trust National Institute for EBP, College of Nursing, Columbus, Ohio, USA

WENDY R. MILLER, PhD, RN, CNS, CCRN, FAAN
Department of Community Health Systems, Indiana University School of Nursing,
Indianapolis, Indiana, USA

MALISSA MULKEY, MSN, APRN, CCNS, CCRN, CNRN
Neuroscience Clinical Nurse Specialist, Advanced Clinical Practice, Duke University
Hospital, Durham, North Carolina, USA

MARSHA NEVILLE, PhD, OTR
Department of Occupational Therapy, School of Occupational Therapy, Texas Woman's
University, Dallas, Texas, USA

DAIWAI M. OLSON, PhD, RN, CCRN, FNCS
Professor, Neurology and Neurotherapeutics, The University of Texas Southwestern
Medical Center, Dallas, Texas, USA

STEFANY ORTEGA-PEREZ, RN, MSc, PhD(c)
Assistant Professor, Nursing Department, Universidad del Norte, Barranquilla,
Colombia

CANDICE L. OSBORNE, PhD, MPH, OTR
Department of Physical Medicine and Rehabilitation, The University of Texas
Southwestern Medical Center, Dallas, Texas, USA

CHRISTINE PICINICH, MS, RN, AGACNP-BC, CCRN
Neurocritical Care Nurse Practitioner, Department of Neurological Surgery, UC Davis
Health, Sacramento, California, USA

AVA M. PUCCIO, RN, PhD
Assistant Professor, Department of Neurological Surgery, Co-Director, Neurotrauma
Clinical Trials Center, University of Pittsburgh, Pittsburgh, Pennsylvania, USA

LORI M. RHUDY, PhD, RN, CNRN, ACNS-BC
Nurse Scientist, Assistant Professor, Department of Nursing, Division of Nursing
Research, Mayo Clinic, Rochester, Minnesota, USA

LORENA SANCHEZ-RUBIO, RN, MSN, PhD(c)
Assistant Professor, Nursing Department, Universidad del Tolima, Ibagué,
Colombia

LALITA R. THOMPSON, MSN, RN, CRRN
Rehabilitation Nurse, TIRR Memorial Hermann, Houston, Texas, USA

MEG ZOMORODI, PhD, RN, CNL
Assistant Provost and Director, Office of Interprofessional Education and Practice, Associate Professor, School of Nursing, The University of North Carolina at Chapel Hill, Chapel Hill, North Carolina, USA

Contents

> The burden of neurologic disease in the United States continues to increase due to a growing older population, increased life expectancy, and improved mortality after cancer and cardiac disease. Emergency medical services (EMS) providers are responding to more patients with stroke, traumatic neurologic injury, neuromuscular weakness, seizure, and spontaneous cardiac arrest. Efficient prehospital care and triage to facilities with specialized services improve outcomes. Effective handoff from EMS to an emergency department ensures continuity of care and patient safety. Although advancements in prehospital cardiopulmonary resuscitation have increased rates of return to spontaneous circulation, a large proportion of patients sustain neurologic injury.

> The neurologic patient presenting to the emergency department is especially complex, with the goal of care being to prevent secondary injury while maximizing oxygenation and perfusion to the brain. To maximize the outcomes for the neurologic patient, the interprofessional team in the ED must be vigilant to ensure that patient transitions occur smoothly. Proactive measures are taken as soon as possible to prevent secondary injury and not delay access to care or services. This article provides an overview of strategies used to assist the ED care team in managing a smooth transition to the next level of care.

> Handoff of patients from the operating room to the intensive care unit is a complex process. It involves 2 teams of caregivers, the physical relocation of the patient and monitoring equipment, and tight time constraints. Research and quality projects have focused on checklists and protocols to standardize handoff processes and content. Interventions also include

requiring all team members be present, a team leader identified, and pre-handoff communication. Outcome evaluation is limited by lack of standardized outcomes to define a good handoff. Instead, handoff content is often used as a proxy. Studies with larger sample sizes using rigorous methods are needed.

Transition of care from the intensive care unit to acute care units after critical neurologic injury includes the consideration of a variety of factors to ensure safe and effective care, and promote ongoing neurologic recovery. Assessment of effectiveness of deescalation techniques, agitation management, and risk factor mitigation are important strategies to enhance the success of transitions. Clear and consistent interdisciplinary communication between teams during hand-off between units is imperative to decrease the risk of complications and errors, and to streamline discharge processes.

Transitions of care from acute hospitalization to postacute rehabilitation settings evolved as a function of cost-saving changes to the Medicare Prospective Payment System. Restricted criteria for inpatient rehabilitation facility admission limited access for patients with severe physical and cognitive deficits. Once used as a resource-intense supplement to hospital care, skilled nursing facilities have metamorphosed into rehabilitation settings with limited nursing staff, lower intensity of therapies, and decreased community discharge rates. A collaborative approach to care transitions, using acute and postacute health care providers, provides the opportunity to improve this process. Early physiatry consultation is a strategy for patients with neurologic disease.

A systematic review of qualitative studies that examined the experience of early supported discharge (ESD) from the perspective of patients with stroke and their caregivers and health care providers revealed an emphasis on psychosocial aspects—the patient-provider relationship, the value of the home environment, and the ability to tailor treatment to meet patient-oriented goals. Patients, caregivers, and providers stressed the importance of clear and systematic communication throughout the ESD process to support transitions, prevent duplication of services, foster trust in relationships, and ensure that patients and caregivers have the knowledge and skills required to manage a chronic condition long term.

Advances in stroke detection and treatment have increased the number of patients discharged home following an index stroke admission. Unfortunately, the science of how to facilitate transition of care (TOC) from hospital to home has not kept pace with decades-long focus on restoring cerebral perfusion. This article examines TOC interventions in stroke populations published after the 2011 Agency for Healthcare Research and Quality report. Early supported discharge is the leading TOC intervention. Diversity of outcome measures and use of poorly defined comparators limits generalizability. There is no clear best practice to define interventions targeted at the hospital to home transition.

Survivors of stroke require long-term follow-up with a focus on rehabilitation, prevention of depression and anxiety, and support for carer. Research is needed in many areas of poststroke care to identify interventions that may ameliorate the sequelae.

The trajectory status of patients with mild, moderate, and severe traumatic brain injury from emergency room evaluation, through acute care (intensive care if severe) and discharge is discussed. Additional considerations for elderly population and common complications associated with severe traumatic brain injury are also covered.

Epilepsy is a complex neurologic disease that requires both medical management and self-management. People with epilepsy and their families complete many transitions throughout the health care system in managing this disease. This article reviews key transitions for people with epilepsy and discusses strategies for improving these transitions.

Dementia is defined as loss of intellectual functions, including thinking, remembering, and reasoning. Cognitive deficits are severe enough to interfere with an individual's daily functioning. Frontotemporal dementia (FTD) is a result of degeneration of the frontal and/or temporal lobes of the brain. FTD is a leading cause of early-onset dementia in approximately 10% of dementia cases. FTD presents in the fourth and fifth decades as progressive changes in personality, affect, and behavior. The etiology of FTD is unknown; treatment focuses on behavioral and symptom

There are roughly 600 million people in the Latin America and the Caribbean region, of whom approximately 36% are living at or below the poverty line. According to this, neurologic injury disorders disproportionately affect this population, which faces not only most risk factors, but also has less developed health systems to deal with illness recovery. Further, most of the risk factors can be attributed to classic preventable cardiovascular risk factors, although there are important differences in demographics, socioeconomic status, and injury mechanisms that may influence the patient's outcome.

NURSING CLINICS OF NORTH AMERICA

FORTHCOMING ISSUES

December 2019
Psychiatric Disorders
Rene Love, *Editor*

March 2020
Building Innovative Nurse Leaders at the Point of Care
Kelly A. Wolgast, *Editor*

June 2020
Orthopedic Nursing
Tandy Gabbert, *Editor*

RECENT ISSUES

June 2019
Infectious Diseases
Randolph F. R. Rasch, *Editor*

March 2019
Quality Improvement
Treasa 'Susie' Leming-Lee and
Richard Watters, *Editors*

December 2018
Nephrology: Innovations in Clinical Practice
Deborah Ellison and Francisca Cisneros
Farrar, *Editors*

SERIES OF RELATED INTEREST

Critical Care Nursing
Available at: https://www.ccnursing.theclinics.com/

THE CLINICS ARE AVAILABLE ONLINE!
Access your subscription at:
www.theclinics.com

Foreword

I Think, Therefore I Am

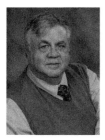

Stephen D. Krau, PhD, RN, CNE
Consulting Editor

I Think, Therefore I Am

When Descartes, the French philosopher and mathematician, first proposed this philosophical stance, his tenet was to provide a foundational stance in the face of radical doubt. In essence, it is an explanation of how we prove beyond a reasonable doubt that something exists. We use our senses of what we see, smell, and hear to provide evidence that something empirically exists. In order to do this, we place our beliefs under the examination of radical doubt. Rather than trying to prove anything beyond reasonable doubt, Descartes proposes that every belief that can be doubted, even beyond conventional reason, does not necessarily form a part of his philosophical foundation. The implications of this for nursing science have far-reaching implications for what we perceive to "know." In fact, the notion provides the basis for our very existence.

Thinking is a primary function of the brain. When there are neurologic issues that impact the brain, our notions, behaviors, and the essence of who we are impacted. So far beyond the philosophical foundation proposed by Descartes, our sense of being or essence of ourselves is impacted. Beyond the philosophical considerations, neurologic disorders are the leading cause of disability and the second leading cause of death worldwide.[1] The number of people dying, or remaining disabled from neurologic disorders, has increased globally over the past 25 years. Often, neurologic disorders are categorized when considering the global burden of a disease as a component of neurologic, mental health, developmental, and substance use. These disorders are expected to rise worldwide, partly because of the projected increase in the numbers of persons who will be at increased risk due to reaching ages in which many disorders occur.[2]

Over the past 20 years, exciting basic science discoveries have been made; effective interventions have been developed, and advances in technology have set the stage for a research agenda that can lead to unprecedented progress in areas of

Nurs Clin N Am 54 (2019) xiii–xiv
https://doi.org/10.1016/j.cnur.2019.06.001
0029-6465/19/© 2019 Published by Elsevier Inc.

nursing.theclinics.com

predicting and treating neurologic disorders.[2] Only through increased engagement among the scientific community, funding agencies for research, global governments, academic institutions, advocacy organizations, and health care professionals can a reduction of disease and disability associated with brain and other nervous system disorders occur. For this to occur, health professionals are tasked with building upon current knowledge of overall neurologic health, toward the goal of improving the lives of those living with brain and other nervous system disorders.[2] Going back to Descartes, we must expand what we know and incorporate this into our professional standards and behaviors.

Stephen D. Krau, PhD, RN, CNE
Vanderbilt University School of Nursing
6809 Highland Park Drive
Nashville, TN 37205, USA

E-mail address:
sbluefountain@aol.com

REFERENCES

1. GBD 2016 Neurology Collaborators, Feigin VL, Nichols E, Alam T, et al. Global, regional, and national burden of neurological disorders, 1990–2016: a systematic analysis for the Global Burden of Disease Study 2016. Lancet Neurol 2019;18: 459–80.
2. Siberberg D, Anand NP, Michels K, et al. Brain and other nervous system disorders across the lifespan-global challenges and opportunities. Nature 2015;527:S151–4.

Preface

Transitions of Care: A New Wave of Research for Patients with Neurologic Diagnoses

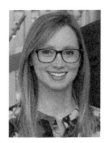

Sonja E. Stutzman, PhD
Editor

Transition is something that everyone experiences. Some transitions can be easy, smooth, and even exciting, like the transition to becoming a new parent or lessening the frequency of your doctor's appointments after being declared in a state of remission. Other transitions are scary, traumatic, or burdensome, like saying good-bye to a loved one, or going to a rehabilitation setting when you were hoping to go home. Whether it's in a medical or nonmedical setting, support and "knowing what to expect" can ease the transition for all involved. I've heard from nurses, patients, physicians, administrators, and loved ones that health-related transitions are oftentimes more stressful than they are calming. There has been a recent movement to enhance transitions within the health care setting by implementing numerous protocols, procedures, and practices in order to decrease risk and burden.

Transitions are rooted in helping someone move from 1 state to another, such as from childhood to adulthood, from independent to dependent living, or from one care area to another. Within the health literature, a transition is considered to be a high-risk time for the patient and the clinician, with adverse events such as medication errors or miscommunication being the primary concern. The word transition, or more specifically the transition of care, has become a buzzword among physicians, nurses, researchers, and administrators, which has propelled a granular dive in to research, protocols, procedures, and evidence-based practice. Recent research has shown that effective communication between clinicians and family members is imperative to creating a smooth transition. Oftentimes, physicians make clinical decisions about the transition of care, but the education provided to the patient and care partners is provided by the nurse. In addition, the summary of the management of the patient's care, and current patient needs are provided from the nurse to another clinician

Nurs Clin N Am 54 (2019) xv–xvi
https://doi.org/10.1016/j.cnur.2019.05.001   **nursing.theclinics.com**
0029-6465/19/© 2019 Published by Elsevier Inc.

(eg, nurse, social worker, care coordinator), making the nurse's role in the transitions of care of utmost importance.

This issue of the *Nursing Clinics of North America* addresses transitions of care for patients with a neurologic diagnosis, including transitions from onset of symptoms through the hospitalization and eventual return to home. Neurologic diagnoses are unique as the road to recovery can be long, with "recovery" looking different for each patient. Furthermore, these patients, and their care partners, experience multiple transitions of care, which does not always follow a linear pattern. We highlight the historical context of transitions as well as the current state of various transitions of care. These transitions in care involve collaboration between clinical teams and patient teams. You will see themes of challenges with communication, addressing roles, and overcoming barriers weaved throughout this issue. In addition, trajectories of transitions of care for specific diseases, such as stroke, traumatic brain injury, seizure disorders, and neurodegenerative disorders, are addressed. A particular focus is placed on the nurse's role within the transition of care, which is extremely important to lessening the patient, family, and clinician strain during this time. Each author has specified successes and areas of improvement within each step of the transition of care to provide nurses with a resource when considering implications for their own practice, procedures, and patient care.

Sonja E. Stutzman, PhD
O'Donnell Brain Institute, University of Texas Southwestern Medical Center
5323 Harry Hines Boulevard
Dallas, TX 75390-8855, USA

E-mail address:
Sonja.Stutzman@UTSouthwestern.edu

Activation to Arrival
Transition and Handoff from Emergency Medical Services to Emergency Departments

Christine Picinich, MS, RN, AGACNP-BC, CCRN[a],*,
Lori Kennedy Madden, PhD, RN, ACNP-BC, CCRN-K, CNRN[b],
Kellie Brendle, RN, MS, CNS[c]

KEYWORDS

- Patient transfer • Emergency medical services (EMS) • Emergency departments (ED)
- Traumatic brain injury (TBI) • Spinal cord injury (SCI) • Stroke • EMS patient handoff

KEY POINTS

- The number of patients with neurologic illness continues to increase, and emergency medical services (EMS) must be prepared to care for this growing patient population.
- Early identification and treatment of neurologic conditions in the prehospital setting improve outcomes.
- Patients with neurologic injury require triage to a hospital with specialized care. The hospital can vary depending on the diagnosis.
- Effective patient handoff from EMS to an emergency department is essential for continuity of care and patient safety.

INTRODUCTION

The burden of neurologic disease in the Unites States continues to increase.[1] A growing older population, increased life expectancy, and improved mortality after cancer and cardiac disease all have contributed to higher rates of stroke and neurodegenerative disease.[2] In 2015, close to 7 million individuals in the United States visited an emergency department (ED) for a neurologic problem.[3] Neurologic disease currently affects more than 100 million Americans, and emergency medical services (EMS)

Disclosure Statement: All authors cite no relationship with any commercial companies that have any direct financial interest in subject matter or materials discussed.
[a] Department of Neurological Surgery, UC Davis Health, 4860 Y Street, Suite 3740, Sacramento, CA 95817, USA; [b] Center for Nursing Science, UC Davis Health, 2315 Stockton Boulevard, Sacramento, CA 95817, USA; [c] Heart and Vascular Services, UC Davis Health, 2315 Stockton Boulevard, Sacramento, CA 95817, USA
* Corresponding author.
E-mail address: cpicinich@ucdavis.edu

must be prepared to care for them as they present for evaluation, treatment, and transport from the prehospital setting to an ED.[2]

Patients with neurologic conditions activating EMS require efficient, specialized care. Early identification and treatment of neurologic conditions, such as stroke and traumatic brain injury (TBI), in the prehospital setting improve outcome.[4,5] Patients with neurologic injury often require neuroscience expertise, and early triage to a center with specialty services is preferred. Prehospital notification and effective patient handoff between EMS and ED care providers are essential for continuity of care and patient safety.[6,7]

TRIAGE, TRANSPORT, AND PATIENT HANDOFF

The EMS providers should assess patients promptly to determine the injury and mechanism.[8] This process, known as field triage, is used to determine where EMS should transfer a patient.[8] This is especially important for patients with severe or life-threatening injury that requires treatment at a Level I or Level II trauma center.[8] The Centers for Disease Control and Prevention (CDC) published "Guidelines for Field Triage of Injured Patients," which includes an algorithm to determine whether a patient requires transfer to a trauma center.[8] Each region should have an organized trauma system and a protocol to determine the appropriate destination facility.[9] It is important to limit time in the field for patients with time-sensitive injury.[10] Patients with severe, life-threatening, or time-critical conditions should be transported via air when ground transport is longer than 45 minutes.[10]

A key element of transition of care from the prehospital setting to an ED is communication between EMS and ED providers. Effective patient handoff is dependent on multiple factors, as outlined in **Table 1**.[11] Patient handoff should include both verbal and written or electronic report from EMS.[6] Pertinent information that should be communicated includes airway status and management, vital signs, neurologic examination, therapeutic interventions, mechanism of injury, time of symptom onset, and relevant medical history.[6,9,10] Responses to or lack of improvement after interventions offered in the field should be reported in handoff. Use of a standardized tool, such as that outlined in **Table 2**, ensures delivery of important information.[12] Results of any diagnostic tests should be provided for the receiving care team.[6] Verbal report, via radio or phone, must include pertinent information so that receiving ED providers can activate necessary facility resources for patients to receive on arrival. Ideally, electronic medical information should be transferred from EMS to the receiving care team in real time.[6] Health systems should work to integrate electronic information from EMS to improve accuracy of patient handoff.[6]

Table 1	
Elements of ideal patient handoff	
Right environment	Quiet; ensures privacy of information, minimal interruptions
Right staff	Appropriate staff available to receive report from EMS; limit repeating report
Right structure	Use of standardized format; information shared in organized and consistent manner
Right time	Report delivered in concise, efficient manner

Table 2
Emergency medical services to emergency department organized patient handoff

Identification	Patient name, age, gender
Chief complaint	Explanation of illness, mechanism of injury
Status	Patient stability, presence of other injuries, interventions performed by bystanders
Assessment	Objective findings on physical examination, vital signs, GCS, pupils, weakness, BE-FAST score
Interventions	Treatment given, patient response
Background	Past medical history, current medications, allergies, other

STROKE

Stroke is a leading cause of disability and the fifth leading cause of death in the United States.[13] Approximately 795,000 Americans suffer a new or recurrent stroke every year. On average, a stroke occurs every 40 seconds and kills approximately 137,000 people a year.[14]

Stroke can be categorized as acute ischemic stroke (AIS), transient ischemic attack (TIA), intracerebral hemorrhage (ICH), or subarachnoid hemorrhage (SAH).[15] AIS and TIA are caused by an embolism from atherosclerosis, small vessel disease, cardiac pathology, and vessel dissection.[16] If no clearly attributable cause is identified, a stroke may be classified as cryptogenic. A TIA stroke is a brief episode with neurologic deficits resulting from focal cerebral ischemia without permanent cerebral infarction but with high likelihood of having a recurrent TIA stroke within 24 hours.[17] Caused by a ruptured blood vessel in the brain, hemorrhagic stroke is classified by its anatomic site or etiology.[16] Hemorrhagic stroke occurs when a blood vessel is weakened and bleeds into the surrounding area of the brain (ICH and SAH). A SAH refers to bleeding within the subarachnoid space and occurs most often because of an aneurysm. A ICH is an intracerebral hemorrhage that can be caused by trauma, aneurysm, or brain tumor. The most common causes, however, are hypertension, cerebral amyloid angiopathy, anticoagulation, and vascular structural lesions.

Stroke patients experience an abrupt onset of focal neurologic deficits or awaken with symptoms. The most common symptoms noted are acute onset of hemiparesis, sudden confusion, headache, facial droop, and trouble with one or more of the following: speaking, seeing in one or both eyes, walking, or balance/coordination. Conditions that mimic a stroke are seizure, migraine headaches, hypoglycemia, dementia, and metabolic syndrome. Providers in EMS and the ED should use the Balance, Eyes, Face, Arm, Speech, and Time (BE-FAST) test to screen for stroke.[16,18] Thorough evaluation of a patient's history and identification of when last known normal (LKN) and completion of the National Institutes of Health Stroke Scale[19] should be accomplished rapidly. On arrival to the receiving facility, noncontrast and contrast CT scans should be completed to rule out an intracranial hemorrhage.[14]

Early EMS stroke recognition and system activation improve stroke detection and facilitate early treatment and arrival to an appropriate stroke center that has neurologic expertise. The decision to transport a patient to a particular hospital or prenotify the hospital is based on a patient's clinical condition.[20] The EMS personnel must be trained to accurately identify patients who are having stroke-like symptoms using a stroke scale, such as the Cincinnati Prehospital Stroke Scale and/or BE-FAST scale.[21] Activating the ED using a prehospital stroke alert system includes report of history and EMS examination findings with stroke assessment to help to alert the stroke team and ready resources, such as CT, pharmacy for thrombolytics, and the neurointerventional team.[20] This results in improved process measures, including metrics that report the notification and timing details, as well as early blood pressure management, airway management, stroke mimic identification, and patient functional outcomes.

The goal for AIS patients is to rapidly reperfuse brain tissue at risk for infarction. Emergency treatment includes CT and CT angiogram to rule out a hemorrhagic stroke, cardiac monitoring, blood pressure management, airway support, and administration of alteplase (tissue plasminogen activator). The administration of alteplase should be given in less than 60 minutes from a patient's arrival or door-to-needle time.[22] Because treatment time for alteplase is within 3 hours of LKN and 4.5 hours for a select group of patients, communication about a patient's LKN from EMS to a receiving facility is an essential part of the handoff. Those patients eligible for intra-arterial alteplase and mechanical thrombectomy due to a middle cerebral artery occlusion need to be treated at a qualified stroke center with access to cerebral angiography and a qualified neurointerventionalist. Updated EMS protocols allow paramedics to transport patients directly to a comprehensive stroke center, where patients have access to a neurointerventionalist.[23]

Prehospital medical management of stroke patients includes a 12-lead ECG, includes placement of two intravenous (IV) catheters, obtaining 12-lead ECG, blood glucose level, vital signs, providing supplemental oxygen, and evaluating for signs of stroke.[24] Some programs include radio communication from the field directly with a neurologist to assess for treatment eligibility based on communication of neurologic examination.[24] The early transmission of patient information allows an ED to assemble the necessary personnel to treat stroke patients.[25] Once a patient arrives at the hospital and neuroimaging is completed, a treatment strategy is made.[24]

Focused history taking from bystanders can help inform definitive care at the receiving hospital. Risk factors for stroke patients can be categorized as modifiable and nonmodifiable.[15] Modifiable risk factors include high blood pressure, atrial fibrillation, smoking, carotid artery disease, methamphetamine use of, street drugs, alcohol, obesity, sleep apnea, smoking, diabetes, and high cholesterol. Nonmodifiable risk factors comprise age, gender, race/ethnicity, and family history. Handoff between EMS and the ED includes communication of any of these pertinent risk factors.

TRAUMATIC NEUROLOGIC INJURY

Traumatic neurologic injury accounts for a large proportion of injury, disability, and death. In 2015, 41.6 million Americans were treated for injuries in EDs, with more than 500,000 patients diagnosed with TBI.[3] On average, 17,700 Americans sustain a new spinal cord injury (SCI) each year.[26] Both TBI and SCI disproportionately affect men, with approximately 78% of new SCIs in males.[26] Fall is the leading cause of nonfatal injury among all age groups and is a common mechanism of traumatic neurologic injury followed by motor vehicle collisions.[27,28] Over the past 30 years, the average age of patients at time of SCI has increased, from 29 in the 1970s to 43 in 2018.[26]

Traumatic Brain Injury

Patients with TBI require immediate field triage and assessment. EMS providers should determine the probability of TBI by assessing for signs of head trauma, depressed skull fracture, high-velocity mechanism, or low Glasgow Coma Scale (GCS) score.[9] A brief history should be obtained by EMS to verify mechanism of trauma, medical comorbidities, and current medications, including any antiplatelet or anticoagulant use.[8,10]

Determining injury severity is an important step in deciding where to transfer a patient with TBI.[8–10] Physical assessment, including vital signs, should be performed promptly by EMS (**Fig. 1**).[10] After evaluation of airway, breathing, and circulation (ABC), EMS should assess neurologic status using the GCS.[9,10] Pupils should be examined, with special notice if they are unequal or nonreactive.[9,10] Patients with GCS less than or equal to 13, hypotension, or respiratory distress are more likely to have a severe injury and should be transferred to the highest level of care within the trauma system.[8,9] Scene time should be limited to 10 minutes or less for patients who are unstable or require surgical intervention.[10]

Because EMS and trauma systems vary based on region, knowledge of local hospitals and protocol for trauma patients is important.[8] Patients with severe TBI require transfer to a facility that can provide CT scanning, neurosurgical intervention, and neuromonitoring.[9] EMS providers should refer to approved protocols within their organized trauma system to select an appropriate destination for patients with TBI.[9,10] Patients with severe or life-threatening injury should be transported via helicopter when ambulance time exceeds 45 minutes.[10] Pertinent history, examination findings, GCS score, pupillary response, vital signs, prehospital interventions, and patient response all should be communicated by EMS to ED providers to ensure continuity of care.[6,10]

Traumatic Spinal Cord Injury

Patients with suspected SCI should be evaluated and immobilized promptly to prevent further neurologic injury.[10] The EMS provider should assess the scene and obtain a brief history to determine the mechanism of injury.[10] Early assessment of ABC should be performed.[10] Resuscitation should be done per standard trauma guidelines.[10] If a

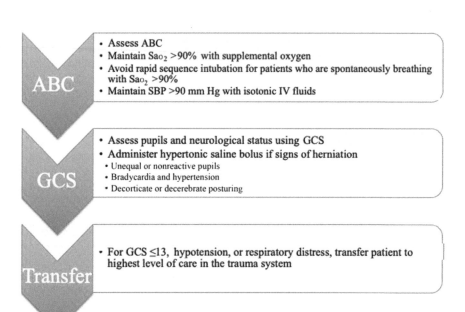

Fig. 1. Suspected traumatic brain injury. Sao2, oxygen saturation; SBP, systolic blood pressure.

patient requires placement of an advanced airway, manual in-line spine stabilization should be used.[29] The patient's mental status should be assessed, along with the presence of neurologic deficit or spinal tenderness.[10]

Transfer to an appropriate center should occur as soon as possible, because delay is associated with worse outcome and increased cost.[30] EMS providers should refer to the CDC "Guidelines for Field Triage of Injured Patients" along with regional trauma system protocol to determine the appropriate destination.[8,10] EMS providers should communicate the GCS score, presence of spinal tenderness or pain, mechanism of injury, extremity weakness, presence of other trauma, prehospital interventions, and pertinent medical history to ED providers.[6,10]

SEIZURE

Approximately 10% of adults experience a seizure in their lifetime. Approximately 1.2% of Americans have active epilepsy, including 3 million adults and 470,000 children.[31,32] Seizures account for 5% to 8% of all EMS calls and 1.2% of ED visits.[33] Status epilepticus, defined as seizure lasting longer than 5 minutes or multiple seizures without return to baseline, has a mortality of 20%.[33] The goal of therapy is to abort both the clinical and electrical seizure activity quickly because early treatment is associated with improved mortality.[34]

Prehospital guidelines recommend initial stabilization of the patient by obtaining a brief history and evaluating ABC and neurologic status.[10,35] EMS' role is to collect history, including identifying the duration of seizure, prior medical history, current medications, recent dose changes or noncompliance, and history of trauma, pregnancy, or toxin exposure.[10] This information helps hospital providers identify the etiology and most appropriate therapy for the seizure.

Initial stabilization should take 5 minutes or less to avoid treatment delay.[34] If a patient continues to actively seize, medications should be administered. Intramuscular administration of midazolam is the first-line EMS treatment of adults and children weighing greater than 40 kg.[10,33,34] After stabilization and initial treatment, patients should be transported to the nearest appropriate medical facility in accordance with local protocol.[8] EMS providers should communicate the following to the ED team: pertinent history, seizure duration, medications given, patient response, GCS, pupillary response, and signs of stroke or other injury.[10]

ACUTE NEUROMUSCULAR WEAKNESS

Weakness is a common nonspecific complaint that may cause individuals to seek evaluation and treatment. Acute-onset weakness may prompt an EMS activation. A variety of conditions can result in generalized fatigue or weakness, such as infection, cardiovascular disease, and dehydration. Differentiating these conditions with underlying neurologic or neuromuscular disease is important, however, for accurate and timely interventions. In the prehospital arena, symptoms associated with neuromuscular weakness are associated most commonly with respiratory insufficiency—specifically, hypoventilation and/or immobility. Life-threatening conditions may cause unilateral or bilateral weakness. During resuscitation, several time-sensitive diagnoses, such as stroke, should be considered.[36] Differentiation of the presentation of weakness may prompt different considerations in treatment. The time frame of onset is important to distinguish (acute, subacute, or chronic) and report to the receiving providers in the ED.

Characterized by rapid-onset muscle weakness, which progresses to maximum severity within several days to weeks (less than 4 weeks), acute neuromuscular paralysis (ANMP) is a common neurologic emergency that requires immediate and careful investigation to determine the etiology because accurate diagnosis has significant impact on therapy and prognosis.[37] Bulbar and respiratory muscle weakness may or may not be present. Respiratory failure caused by neuromuscular weakness may be insidious or subtle until sudden decompensation leads to hypoventilation and life-threatening hypoxia. Although a full history of symptom progression is not within the scope or priority of EMS care, any information obtained from patients and bystanders is valuable in handoff to providers of definitive care. Specifically, the requirement for respiratory support and response to interventions provided prior to and during EMS care should evaluated and reported to the receiving facility.

Generally, ANMP is classified based on the site of defect in motor unit pathway. Identification of the cause is based primarily on history and detailed clinical examination and supplemented with imaging, neurophysiologic testing, and laboratory studies. Brief history and neurologic examination should be focused on onset, progression, pattern, and severity of muscle weakness in the field. Once transferred to a receiving facility, further examination, including cranial nerve testing and tests for autonomic dysfunction, should be done. Observation and report of associated nonneurological features like fever, rash or other skin lesions should be noted by EMS and reported in handoff to ED providers.

Occurring in approximately 1 to 2 people per 100,000 annually, Guillain-Barré syndrome (GBS) is the most frequent cause of ANMP and accounts for the majority of cases of respiratory muscles weakness associated with neuromuscular disorders.[38,39] ANMP is frequently identified in the critical care literature in the context of critical illness polyneuropathy, critical illness myopathy, and drug-induced neuromuscular weakness. Polio virus and West Nile virus (WNV) infections are 2 important causes of infection-associated acute muscular paralysis. Acute, flaccid, and asymmetric motor weakness may occur due to WNV.[40] Although most WNV infections are asymptomatic, fewer than 1% of patients develop more extensive disease, including meningitis, encephalitis, and acute flaccid paralysis. Bulbar and respiratory muscles involvement may occur. History and progression of any report of illness or malaise should be noted by EMS and reported at bedside handoff to the ED.

Although it is rare, GBS patients often presents with a chief complaint of weakness. Also referred to as Landry ascending paralysis, postinfectious polyneuropathy, and acute inflammatory demyelinating polyneuropathy, GBS is a progressive paralyzing disorder of the peripheral nerves. As with many conditions, early consideration is important to provide a better outcome, because delayed treatment can lead to unrecognized failing respiration and life-threatening dysrhythmias. Prehospital care requires careful attention to ABC. Administration of oxygen and assisted ventilation may be indicated, along with establishment of IV access. Approximately one-third of GBS patients require intubation and mechanical ventilation.[41] Local EMS airway management protocols should be followed. Reports of response to interventions provided by EMS and ventilatory effort are essential aspects to include in reports to the receiving facility.

CARDIAC ARREST

Sudden cardiac arrest happens without warning and is the leading cause of death in the United States and developing countries. Approximately 500,000 deaths occur annually in the United States and Europe.[42] There also is a high risk for neurologic disability among cardiac arrest survivors.[42] Advances in prehospital care have improved the rates of return of spontaneous circulation, with more than 60,000 patients being treated in the hospital.[43]

Even with well-performed successful cardiopulmonary resuscitation, cardiac arrest results in insufficient cerebral perfusion and associated brain injury.[44] Stasis of blood in the cerebral vasculature results in the formation of microthrombi.[45] During the time of hypoperfusion, glucose and ATP are not delivered to the brain, resulting in intracellular acidosis. There is disruption of the blood-brain barrier and neuronal edema that also occur, which contribute toward cell death and brain injury.

The American Heart Association offers guidelines to improve survival and recovery of patients who have suffered cardiac arrest.[44] The chain of survival, which starts with public recognition and initiation of treatment of cardiac events and 911 activation of EMS, is inherently reliant on the work of EMS to provide care and handoff of victims to postarrest care at a receiving facility.[44] Prehospital stabilization of sudden cardiac arrest patients includes securing an airway, managing ventilation and oxygenation, preventing hypotension, and elevating the head of the bed to decrease cerebral edema. Treatment goals include titration of supplemental oxygen to keep oxygen saturation as measured by pulse oximetry (Spo_2) greater or equal to 94%, maintain minute ventilation to sustain $Paco_2$ 40 mm Hg to 45 mm Hg, and maintain systolic blood pressure greater than 90 mm Hg.[44,46]

The EMS handoff to an ED can be a complex process where information can be altered or lost.[47] EMS can have multiple different reports in the transition of care that include prehospital reports to ED, triage nurse, and bedside nurse. Communication can be difficult due to interruptions, multitasking, workload, and working relations.[47,48] Utilization of a transition of care tool that ensures accurate patient information, continuity of care, and patient safety improves patient care.[47,48] The handoff may include prehospital report of chief concern, initial presentation, vital signs, age, and overall assessment and may vary from provider to provider.

SUMMARY

Prehospital expertise in the evaluation and care of neurologic illness and injury can make a significant impact on quality and likelihood of survival. Most conditions rely on rapid assessment of the context of presentation (history and related events), quick evaluation, and careful delivery of essential treatment common across conditions. Assessment of patient history includes identifying onset and pattern of weakness, associated symptoms, prior medical history, current medications, and history of recent illness or toxin exposure.[10] Shortness of breath, abnormal respiratory rate and/or effort, use of accessory muscles, abnormal color, and evidence of hypoxemia may be present. Noninvasive ventilation techniques may be implemented and sufficiently provide support. Supplemental oxygen may be administered in the prehospital setting to maintain Spo_2.[10] For impending respiratory failure, varied positive airway pressure techniques may be implemented. If ventilation is compromised, bag-valve-mask ventilation may be used in the setting of respiratory failure. Assessments of ABC remain priorities along with rapid transport to definitive care. After stabilization and initial treatment, patients should be transported to the nearest hospital. The EMS providers should communicate pertinent history, interventions provided, and neurologic and respiratory status. An effective standardized handoff from EMS to receiving team is imperative to patient safety and continuity of care.[12]

REFERENCES

1. Fineberg HV. The state of health in the United States. JAMA 2013;310(6):585-6.

2. Gooch CL, Pracht E, Borenstein AR. The burden of neurological disease in the United States: a summary report and call to action. Ann Neurol 2017;81(4): 479–84.
3. Rui P, Kang K. National hospital ambulatory medical care survey; 2015. Available at: https://www.cdc.gov/nchs/ahcd/web_tables.htm. Accessed October 9, 2018.
4. Bernard SA, Nguyen V, Cameron P, et al. Prehospital rapid sequence intubation improves functional outcome for patients with severe traumatic brain injury: a randomized controlled trial. Ann Surg 2010;252(6):959–65.
5. Fassbender K, Balucani C, Walter S, et al. Streamlining of prehospital stroke management: the golden hour. Lancet Neurol 2013;12(6):585–96.
6. American College of Emergency Physicians, Emergency Nurses Association, National Association of EMS Physicians, National Association of Emergency Medical Technicians, National Association of State EMS Officials. Transfer of patient care between EMS providers and receiving facilities. Prehosp Emerg Care 2014;18(2):305.
7. Goldberg SA, Porat A, Strother CG, et al. Quantitative analysis of the content of EMS handoff of critically ill and injured patients to the emergency department. Prehosp Emerg Care 2017;21(1):14–7.
8. Sasser SM, Hunt RC, Faul M, et al. Guidelines for field triage of injured patients: recommendations of the National Expert Panel on Field Triage, 2011. MMWR Recomm Rep 2012;61(RR-1):1–20.
9. Badjatia N, Carney N, Crocco TJ, et al. Guidelines for prehospital management of traumatic brain injury 2nd edition. Prehosp Emerg Care 2008;12(Suppl 1):S1–52.
10. NASEMSO. National model EMS clinical guidelines. NASEMSO MedicalDirectors Council; 2017. Available at: https://nasemso.org/wp-content/uploads/National-Model-EMS-Clinical-Guidelines.
11. Cheung DS, Kelly JJ, Beach C, et al. Improving handoffs in the emergency department. Ann Emerg Med 2010;55(2):171–80.
12. Meisel ZF, Shea JA, Peacock NJ, et al. Optimizing the patient handoff between emergency medical services and the emergency department. Ann Emerg Med 2015;65(3):310–7.e1.
13. Prabhakaran S, Ruff I, Bernstein RA. Acute stroke intervention: a systematic review. JAMA 2015;313(14):1451–62.
14. Medoro I, Cone DC. An analysis of EMS and ED detection of stroke. Prehosp Emerg Care 2017;21(4):476–80.
15. Yew KS, Cheng EM. Diagnosis of acute stroke. Am Fam Physician 2015;91(8): 528–36.
16. Hankey GJ. Stroke. Lancet 2017;389(10069):641–54.
17. Easton JD, Saver JL, Albers GW, et al. Definition and evaluation of transient ischemic attack: a scientific statement for healthcare professionals from the American Heart Association/American Stroke Association Stroke Council; Council on Cardiovascular Surgery and Anesthesia; Council on Cardiovascular Radiology and Intervention; Council on Cardiovascular Nursing; and the Interdisciplinary Council on Peripheral Vascular Disease. The American Academy of Neurology affirms the value of this statement as an educational tool for neurologists. Stroke 2009;40(6):2276–93.
18. Aroor S, Singh R, Goldstein LB. BE-FAST (balance, eyes, face, arm, speech, time): reducing the proportion of strokes missed using the FAST mnemonic. Stroke 2017;48(2):479–81.
19. Brott T, Adams HP Jr, Olinger CP, et al. Measurements of acute cerebral infarction: a clinical examination scale. Stroke 1989;20(7):864–70.

20. Zhang S, Zhang J, Zhang M, et al. Prehospital notification procedure improves stroke outcome by shortening onset to needle time in chinese urban area. Aging Dis 2018;9(3):426–34.

21. Abboud ME, Band R, Jia J, et al. Recognition of stroke by EMS is associated with improvement in emergency department quality measures. Prehosp Emerg Care 2016;20(6):729–36.

22. Jauch EC, Saver JL, Adams HP Jr, et al. Guidelines for the early management of patients with acute ischemic stroke: a guideline for healthcare professionals from the American Heart Association/American Stroke Association. Stroke 2013;44(3):870–947.

23. DiBiasio EL, Jayaraman MV, Oliver L, et al. Emergency medical systems education may improve knowledge of pre-hospital stroke triage protocols. J Neurointerv Surg 2018.

24. Drenck N, Viereck S, Baekgaard JS, et al. Pre-hospital management of acute stroke patients eligible for thrombolysis - an evaluation of ambulance on-scene time. Scand J Trauma Resusc Emerg Med 2019;27(1):3.

25. Schwamm LH, Chumbler N, Brown E, et al. Recommendations for the implementation of telehealth in cardiovascular and stroke care: a policy statement from the American Heart Association. Circulation 2017;135(7):e24–44.

26. National spinal cord injury statistical center, facts and figures at a glance. Birmingham (AL): University of Alabama at Birmingham; 2019. Available at: https://www.nscisc.uab.edu/Public/Facts%20and%20Figures%20-%202018.pdf.

27. Leading causes of non-fatal injury reports. CDC; 2018. Available at: https://webappa.cdc.gov/sasweb/ncipc/nfilead.html. Accessed 2018.

28. Taylor CA, Bell JM, Breiding MJ, et al. Traumatic brain injury-related emergency department visits, hospitalizations, and deaths - United States, 2007 and 2013. MMWR Surveill Summ 2017;66(9):1–16.

29. Ahn H, Singh J, Nathens A, et al. Pre-hospital care management of a potential spinal cord injured patient: a systematic review of the literature and evidence-based guidelines. J Neurotrauma 2011;28(8):1341–61.

30. Theodore N, Aarabi B, Dhall SS, et al. Transportation of patients with acute traumatic cervical spine injuries. Neurosurgery 2013;72(Suppl 2):35–9.

31. Zack MM, Kobau R. National and state estimates of the numbers of adults and children with active epilepsy - United States, 2015. MMWR Morb Mortal Wkly Rep 2017;66(31):821–5.

32. Cui W, Kobau R, Zack MM, et al. Seizures in children and adolescents aged 6-17 years - United States, 2010-2014. MMWR Morb Mortal Wkly Rep 2015;64(43):1209–14.

33. Silverman EC, Sporer KA, Lemieux JM, et al. Prehospital care for the adult and pediatric seizure patient: current evidence-based recommendations. West J Emerg Med 2017;18(3):419–36.

34. Glauser T, Shinnar S, Gloss D, et al. Evidence-based guideline: treatment of convulsive status epilepticus in children and adults: report of the guideline committee of the American Epilepsy Society. Epilepsy Curr 2016;16(1):48–61.

35. Billington M, Kandalaft OR, Aisiku IP. Adult status epilepticus: a review of the pre-hospital and emergency department management. J Clin Med 2016;5(9) [pii:E74].

36. Flower O, Wainwright MS, Caulfield AF. Emergency neurological life support: acute non-traumatic weakness. Neurocrit Care 2015;23(Suppl 2):S23–47.

37. Nayak R. Practical approach to the patient with acute neuromuscular weakness. World J Clin Cases 2017;5(7):270–9.

38. Ropper AH. The Guillain-Barre syndrome. N Engl J Med 1992;326(17):1130–6.
39. Hutchinson D, Whyte K. Neuromuscular disease and respiratory failure. Pract Neurol 2008;8(4):229–37.
40. Carson PJ, Borchardt SM, Custer B, et al. Neuroinvasive disease and West Nile virus infection, North Dakota, USA, 1999-2008. Emerg Infect Dis 2012;18(4): 684–6.
41. Yuki N, Hartung HP. Guillain-Barre syndrome. N Engl J Med 2012;366(24): 2294–304.
42. Girotra S, Chan PS, Bradley SM. Post-resuscitation care following out-of-hospital and in-hospital cardiac arrest. Heart 2015;101(24):1943–9.
43. Elmer J, Polderman KH. Emergency neurological life support: resuscitation following cardiac arrest. Neurocrit Care 2017;27(Suppl 1):134–43.
44. Koenig MA. Brain resuscitation and prognosis after cardiac arrest. Crit Care Clin 2014;30(4):765–83.
45. Madl C, Holzer M. Brain function after resuscitation from cardiac arrest. Curr Opin Crit Care 2004;10(3):213–7.
46. Peberdy MA, Callaway CW, Neumar RW, et al. Part 9: post-cardiac arrest care: 2010 American Heart Association guidelines for cardiopulmonary resuscitation and emergency cardiovascular care. Circulation 2010;122(18 Suppl 3):S768–86.
47. Reay G, Norris JM, Alix Hayden K, et al. Transition in care from paramedics to emergency department nurses: a systematic review protocol. Syst Rev 2017; 6(1):260.
48. Bost N, Crilly J, Patterson E, et al. Clinical handover of patients arriving by ambulance to a hospital emergency department: a qualitative study. Int Emerg Nurs 2012;20(3):133–41.

Time is Brain
Setting Neurologic Patients Up for Success from Emergency Department to Hospital Admission

Meg Zomorodi, PhD, RN, CNL[a],*,
Megan A. Brissie, DNP, RN, ACNP-BC, CEN[b]

KEYWORDS

- Care transition • Emergency departments • Transfer of care • Safety
- Communication

KEY POINTS

- The spectrum of neurologic emergencies that are encountered in the Emergency Department (ED) is wide and treatment modalities are evolving at a rapid pace.
- The role of the ED nurse is to prevent secondary neurologic injury and stabilize the patient for an appropriate transfer out of the ED.
- The neurologic examination is the most pressing need for the ED nurse to complete on the patient's arrival, as this determines the diagnostic and treatment course.
- An effective handoff is essential to maintain the quality of the care transition from ED to hospital for the neurologic patient.

INTRODUCTION

Patients with life-threatening or potentially life-threatening neurologic conditions often enter through the Emergency Department (ED). Every year more than 136 million people in the United States visit the ED annually.[1] Although reasons may vary, most ED visits consist of (1) lack of a primary care provider; (2) an aging United States population; (3) hospital readmissions; (4) acute mental health crises; (5) lack of access to care, including ED closures nationally; and (6) lack of adequate health insurance.[1] Neurologic patients encompass all of these reasons for visiting the ED and can range from acute need to chronic management.[2] Neurologic emergencies in the ED constitute approximately 10% to 15% of all medical emergencies.[3]

Disclosure Statement: The authors have nothing to disclose.
[a] Office of Interprofessional Education and Practice, School of Nursing, The University of North Carolina at Chapel Hill, CB# 7460, Carrington Hall, Chapel Hill, NC 27599-7470, USA;
[b] Department of Neurosurgery, Duke University Health System, Duke Regional Hospital, 3643 North Roxboro Road, Durham, NC 27704, USA
* Corresponding author.
E-mail address: Meg_Zomorodi@unc.edu

The spectrum of neurologic emergencies that are encountered in the ED is wide and treatment modalities are evolving at a rapid pace. Some common life-threatening neurologic emergencies seen in the ED include, but are not limited to, traumatic brain injury (TBI), acute ischemic stroke, aneurysmal subarachnoid hemorrhage (aSAH), intracranial hemorrhage, and seizures. Accurate diagnosis is critical in these patients because many treatments are time dependent and crucial to the patients' long-term outcome.[4] Incorrect or delayed diagnosis can result in neurologic damage and poor clinical outcomes, and delay appropriate treatment; all the while making care for the neurologic patient in the ED especially challenging. Owing to the variety of neurologic conditions that the ED faces, many nurses often feel ill-prepared to care for the neurologic patient. The role of the ED nurse is to identify life-threatening injuries, secure and maintain the patient's airway, breathing, and circulation, prevent secondary neurologic injury, and stabilize the patient for an appropriate transfer out of the ED. Transferring out of the ED might include a rapid transition to the intensive care unit (ICU), admission to the acute inpatient unit within the facility, preparing the patient for emergency surgery, or transferring the patient to a higher level of care at another institution. The complexities of the neurologic patient can make these care transitions especially difficult.

Transitions of care are defined as the "movement of patients between health care practitioners, settings, and home as their condition and care needs change."[5] Every patient deserves to have their care transition go smoothly, but this is not always the case. Root causes of ineffective care transitions include (1) miscommunication, (2) lack of patient education, and (3) breakdowns in accountability and fragmentation of care.[6] For these reasons, transitions of care must be interprofessional and involve every member of the care team in the ED. This will often include the bedside nurse caring for the patient, the ED physician, the ED charge nurse, the neurologist or neurosurgeon evaluating and/or admitting the patient, and the accepting nurse on the inpatient unit or in the operating room. When a patient is being transferred to a higher level of care, hospital policies are in place to ensure a safe patient transition. The Emergency Medical Treatment and Labor Act is a federal law that ensures all patients are cared for and stabilized in the ED before being transferred to another institution, regardless of their ability to pay.[7]

Institutions at Level 1 trauma centers often will have a transfer center to assist with accepting new patients into their hospital system. This facilitates ease of patient movement, allows for clear communication to the accepting physician, and provides an opportunity for safe handoff between nursing staff. Ground or air transport is often arranged via a centralized transfer center to assist with prompt transfer of acutely ill patients. Through such established collaborative relationships between all members of the care team, accountability is shared, resulting in better handoffs and reduced fragmentation of care. Interventions, such as having printed handoff tools and care plan notes that engage patients as active participants in this process, have shown stronger shared accountability, safer handovers, stronger communication, and lower rehospitalization rates.[8,9] The purpose of this article is to provide an overview of these strategies to assist the ED care team in managing these care transitions to ensure a smooth transition to the next level of care.

TYPES OF EMERGENCY DEPARTMENTS AND GOALS FOR NEUROLOGIC SERVICES

In the United States there are 3 levels of emergency services: primary (Level 1), secondary (Level 2), and tertiary (Level 3). In a Level 1 trauma center, the ED is able to give definitive, rapid care for all critical emergency situations, and is usually part of an academic or teaching hospital.[10] Level 1 trauma centers are equipped for poly-level traumas including traumatic brain injuries, subarachnoid hemorrhages, status epilepticus, and spinal cord injury. Level I trauma centers are staffed with 24-hour access to in-house trauma surgeons and on-call specialists, and provide access to advanced neurologic imaging and neurologic specialist services including neurology and neurosurgery. Care transitions for these patients can include resources within the same hospital, including emergent access to operating rooms, advanced diagnostic imaging, and high-acuity specialty ICUs. In addition, Level 1 trauma centers are usually associated with a teaching hospital and are staffed by resident and fellow physicians, along with other health care professionals in training. Resources within the hospital are typically available 24 hours a day, including diagnostic testing and imaging, to assist with the care of complex critical patients.

Level 2 (secondary ED) can care for most neurologic emergencies and have specialists on call and available within 1 hour. A Level 2 ED can manage new-onset seizures, concussions, new diagnosis of tumors, meningitis management, and workup for most acute neurologic injuries. In these situations, the ED intervenes for the patient until the specialist is available to transition the care to the appropriate provider or institution. Level 3 (tertiary centers) do not have all specialists available, and care is focused on stabilizing the patient and transferring them to the appropriate care facility as needed. In all of these cases, assessment skills and documentation are critical to help establish history of the present illness and baseline assessments.

There are 2 types of stroke centers in the United States: primary stroke centers and comprehensive stroke centers. For the neurologic patient exhibiting signs of an acute ischemic stroke (B.E. F.A.S.T.: balance abnormalities, blurry vision, facial weakness, arm weakness, speech abnormalities, and time), the patient should be transferred to either a primary stoke center or, ideally, a comprehensive stroke center.[11] These centers are certified by the Joint Commission, and are equipped to quickly perform the necessary computed tomography scan and neurologic examinations. As treatment recommendations continue to evolve for ischemic strokes, both primary and comprehensive stroke centers are best equipped to administer the clot-busting medication, intravenous (IV) alteplase. Alteplase can stop or reverse the signs of stroke when given within the recommended time frame of 3 to 4.5 hours. In addition, comprehensive stroke centers are also equipped with neurointerventionalists who have the ability to directly retrieve the clot in those patients who meet criteria up to 6 hours after symptom onset. Comprehensive stroke centers provide extensive evaluation in the acute time frame following the onset of stroke.[12] These centers must have intensive care beds available to care for these patients and have experts in place to meet the detailed care management, coordination, and rehabilitation services necessary following stroke.

GOALS FOR NEUROLOGIC MANAGEMENT

The goals for ED management of the neurologic patient are to stabilize and prevent secondary injury. In traumatic brain injuries, secondary injury occurs after the initial injury and results in a reduction of oxygenation and perfusion to the brain. In the stroke patient, a lack of oxygen can occur when there is an ischemic event (embolic or thrombotic clot) or hemorrhagic stroke (subarachnoid hemorrhage or ruptured vessel).[13] For other neurologic events, a reduction of oxygen can occur because of increased intracranial pressure (ICP).

Increased ICP is potentially life threatening and can occur for a variety of reasons including swelling of the brain resulting from tumor or edema, hydrocephalus (or buildup of the fluid component of the brain) or blockage of the ventricles, a change in blood flow (TBI or thrombus), and changes in metabolic demand such as seizures or infection. Elevated ICP is clinically significant because it diminishes cerebral perfusion pressure (CPP), increases risks of brain ischemia (lack of blood flow) and/or infarction (no blood flow), and is associated with an increased morbidity and mortality.[13]

Although few neurologic patients presenting to the ED will present in these conditions, it is important for the ED team to be vigilant for signs of increasing ICP. Early signs of increasing ICP that the ED nurse should monitor for include headache, active vomiting, or a change in mental status including the patient becoming increasingly more confused, restless, or drowsy. Late signs of increased ICP include unequal or dilated nonreactive pupils, the patient becoming difficult to arouse or unresponsive, or a change in their motor examination, specifically abnormal flexion and extension, or no response to painful stimuli.[14] The ED nurse needs to closely monitor for signs of the Cushing triad, which includes sudden bradycardia, a widening pulse pressure or hypertension, and an irregular respiratory pattern.[15] Strong assessment skills and rapid triage are integral for the appropriate care management and transitions of care for the neurologic patient. The patient, family, and other members of the interprofessional team should be included at every level of transition in the ED from triage, assessment, diagnosis, and transfer within and to another hospital.

For all neurologic issues in the ED, the patient and family should be included in the triage assessment when available. The family and/or patient can be helpful in providing past medical and family history, current list of medications, history of present illness including a review of symptoms, and information about symptom onset. The nurse is responsible for documenting this information in the electronic medical record (EMR) and updating the patient and family regarding transition of care. Having this information established before transfer from the ED can expedite neurologic interventions. Several studies have correlated strong communication skills such as reassuring the family, providing emotional support, listening, encouraging communication, and providing frequent status updates to the patient and family with increased patient outcomes, reduction in ED resource use, and increased patient satisfaction.[16] In addition, as part of the triage assessment, the nurse should ask questions to determine a recent history of falls and last oral intake, and complete a review of current medications including anticoagulants, antiplatelets, and herbal medications to ensure clear documentation is in place, ultimately providing quality care and improved outcomes.

Admission to the Emergency Department

Once the patient has been triaged or has arrived from Emergency Medical Services to the ED, the interprofessional team should be prepared to complete interventions that expedite diagnosis and treatment. Establishing standardized protocols should be used to facilitate diagnoses and reduce the time to treatment for the neurologic patient.

The neurologic examination is the most pressing need for the ED nurse to complete on the patient's arrival, because following a neurologic event this assessment sets the baseline examination and determines the diagnostic and treatment course. Throughout the patient's time in the ED, the ED nurse needs to carefully monitor the patient's neurologic examination because the patient with neurologic injury is at highest risk of declining while in the ED before transfer.[17]

Vital Signs and Blood Pressure Management

To appropriately maximize CPP and reduce the risk of secondary injury, blood pressure should be controlled within prescribed parameters based on the neurologic injury. For example, in the patient is suspected of having an ischemic stroke, treatment options may be limited until blood pressure (BP) is within desired treatment parameters set by the neurologist (systolic BP [SBP] <185 and diastolic BP <110). To prevent hemorrhage expansion in the case of an intracranial hemorrhage (SBP <140) or rerupture of an aSAH (SBP <160) in an unsecured subarachnoid hemorrhage, BP parameters need to be tightly controlled.[18–20] In most cases, SBP is the preferred BP measurement over mean arterial pressure and is recommended to be treated based on the specific disease process.[21,22] Being aware of the recommended treatment parameters to maintain, and notifying the provider when goals are not able to be achieved should be a priority of the ED nurse in order to optimize patient outcomes and prevent complications such as hemorrhage expansion, aneurysm rerupture, seizure, herniation, and death. During IV alteplase administration, the ED nurse must frequently assess the patient (as per health system protocol from time of alteplase initiation) for possible hemorrhage, and work with the interprofessional team to communicate the treatment plan to ensure successful transition from the ED to ICU.

Hemorrhagic Stroke Patients

For patients with a hemorrhagic stroke, it is important to reduce hypertension and prevent further hemorrhage expansion. Depending on the size, location, and type of hemorrhage, the ED nurse might be preparing the patient for possible transition to the operating room to evacuate the clot burden, drain placement, or medical management. If the hemorrhagic stroke is due to an aSAH, the ED team should prepare the patient for intravascular care and/or operating room management, based on the hospital's protocol. In some cases, patients with aSAH may need to be transferred to a higher level of care to appropriately treat their more complex needs. The nurse's role in facilitating a smooth transition from the ED to the next level of care is based on timely transitions of care, strict neurologic assessment, maintenance of the patient's airway and breathing, strict BP management as determined by the neurologic specialists, and monitoring for early and late signs of increasing ICP.

Seizures

Seizure medications should be administered prophylactically for the patient considered at risk for seizures from neurologic irritation caused by hemorrhage, regardless of seizure history. This will often include those patients with an unsecured aSAH who are at risk for rerupture and those patients with a severe TBI. A patient who is experiencing seizures will often have a delay of care during transfer, further increasing the risk of cerebral damage caused by secondary injury and death. When a patient experiences a seizure, the nurse should be vigilant in documenting this assessment; describing the last seizure activity including the time, description, and interventions completed during the seizure event. A full list of medications given should also be provided.

Antibiotics

Antibiotic administration for infection control should also be initiated in the ED by the nurse for patients suspected of neurologic infections, such as meningitis. Careful timing of antibiotic administration needs to be considered once a lumbar puncture is planned and completed and a cerebral spinal fluid sample is obtained. This is important to prevent medication toxicity and to ensure that the antibiotic is given in an appropriate window of time to maximize effectiveness. Failure to communicate this could result in a delay of care; the antibiotic should be given as soon as possible from obtaining the sample to prevent the risk of developing meningitis. Antibiotic management should be continued throughout the transfer process according to the appropriate treatment regimen.

Aspiration Prevention

A recent study found that swallowing impairment occurs in up to 78% of patients with acute stroke, and early screening and implementation of proper feeding strategies and treatment have been linked to better outcomes and decreased risk of aspiration pneumonia.[22] The American Heart Association/American Stroke Association now recommends screening of swallowing before the administration of food, liquid, or medication in individuals presenting with stroke symptoms in the ED.[23] Establishing a swallow-screening protocol helps identify patients who are at risk for dysphagia and can decrease the risk for aspiration. There are several swallowing assessment protocols that have been developed and tested in the ED.[24,25] Establishing a nurse-driven swallowing evaluation assessment can help reduce aspiration, which is a further complication that could delay discharge and increase the length of stay in hospital.

Nasogastric Tubes and Foley Catheters

Insertion of a nasogastric feeding tube should be cautiously considered in the neurologic patient while in the ED before transfer, especially for those patients at risk for aspiration who have a facial droop or tongue deviation at the time of presentation, are dysarthic, aphasic, and may not be able to safely swallow medications or eat without the risk of aspiration. In addition, owing to the high risk of infection from prolonged catheter use, a Foley catheter may or may not need to be urgently inserted in the ED if there are alternative means for safely monitoring urinary output. However, if there is a concern that a patient may not be able to safely swallow or void without the insertion of a nasogastric tube or Foley catheter and will be receiving IV alteplase, ED nurses should consider inserting either or both of these tubes before starting any antithrombotics. This is an important consideration because both Foley catheters and nasogastric tubes should not be established in the first 24 hours after IV alteplase has been initiated because of the increased risk of bleeding. Failure to complete these insertions before IV alteplase administration when the opportunity is available can delay necessary nutritional supplementation and medication administration, and increase the incidence of falls if a patient attempts to get out of bed to void and falls as a result of the new neurologic deficit. The nurses' assessment of these events should be clearly documented in the EMR and communicated as part of the reporting process for transfer from the ED to the ICU.

Communication Handoff and Transfer

Once the plan for the patient has been established by the accepting hospital team, the ED team must prepare the patient for transfer. In one study, 80% of medical errors involved miscommunication during the handoff transition between health care providers.[26,27] The Council of Residency Directors survey reported that more than half of the respondents from academic EDs indicated that their EDs use a standardized handoff. However, it is not known how emergency medicine residency programs are providing training around care transitions from the ED to inpatient settings.[28] In a survey of ED residency programs (n = 121), 74.4% of respondents indicated that handoff training did occur in residency programs, although 48.8% indicated that they do not formally assess the competency of physician handoffs.[28] More research is needed to determine the barriers to effective handoffs in the ED and its impact on patient safety.[29] Some institutions have implemented a resident handoff bundle consisting of training, protocols, and a handoff structure that has been shown to be effective in reducing handoff miscommunications.[30]

A systematic review of handoffs from the ED recommended future research to establish both interprofessional and interdiscipline specific handoff tools that are incorporated in the EMR. By focusing on the EMR, more structured formats can improve the consistency of data shared, increase interprofessional communication, and improve shared accountability.[31] Collins and colleagues'[31] use of the Continuity of Care Document provides a nice framework as a way to establish consistent handoff and handover techniques, although more implementation research is warranted.

SUMMARY

Ineffective care transitions from the ED to the hospital are often effected by poor communication, care fragmentation, the need for patient and family communication, and a breakdown of accountability. This article provides strategies to address these root causes and offers strategies for future work in implementation science and research. More work is needed in all of these areas, especially how the nurse's role in communication affects care transitions. Many of the interventions are focused on medical training, so there is an opportunity for nursing research in this area, especially as it relates to how miscommunication can lead to care fragmentation, handoffs in care, and breakdown of accountability across the care team.[32] Future work can also focus on developing patient and family education materials because this was identified as a gap that needs to be addressed in order to improve care transitions in the ED and ensure that patients and families obtain the high-quality neurologic care they deserve.

REFERENCES

1. Centers for Disease Control and Prevention. National hospital ambulatory medical care survey. 2011. Available at: www.cdc.gov/nchs/faststats/emergency-deprtment.html. Accessed December 28, 2018.
2. Hansen C, Fisher J, Joyce N, et al. A prospective evaluation of indications for neurological consultation in the emergency department. Int J Emerg Med 2015; 8(26). https://doi.org/10.1186/s12245-015-0074-3.
3. Soto V, Morales I, Vega C, et al. Waiting times for neurological emergencies in an emergency room. Rev Med Chil 2018;146(7):885–9.
4. Lees KR, Bluhmki E, von Kummer R, et al. Time to treatment with intravenous alteplase and outcome in stroke: an updated pooled analysis of ECASS, ATLANTIS, NINDS, and EPITHET trials. Lancet 2010;375(9727):1695–703.
5. The Care Transitions Program. Available at: http://www.caretransitions.org/definitions.asp. Accessed December 29, 2018.
6. The Joint Commission. Hot topics in transitions of care. 2012. Available at: https://www.jointcommission.org/assets/1/18/Hot_Topics_Transitions_of_Care.pdf. Accessed December 29, 2018.
7. Centers for Medicare & Medicaid Services. Emergency Medical Treatment & Labor Act (EMTALA). 2012. Available at: CMS.gov. https://www.cms.gov/Regulations-and-Guidance/Legislation/EMTALA/index.html. Accessed December 31, 2018.
8. Hansagi H, Olsson M, Hussain A, et al. Is information sharing between the emergency department and primary care useful to the care of frequent emergency department users? Eur J Emerg Med 2008;15:34–9.

9. Flink M, Ohlen G, Hansagi H, et al. Beliefs and experiences can influence patient participation in handover between primary and secondary care—a qualitative study of patient perspectives. Br Med J 2012;21(1):73–83.

10. American Trauma Center. Trauma center levels explained. Available at: https://www.amtrauma.org/page/TraumaLevels. Accessed December 29, 2018.

11. Aroor S, Singh R, Goldstein L. BE-FAST (balance, eyes, face, arm, speech, time): reducing the proportion of strokes missed using the FAST mnemonic. Stroke 2017;48:417–9.

12. Rehani B, Zhang Y, Ammanuel S, et al. Imaging in neurointerventional stroke treatment: review of the recent trials and what your neurointerventionalist wants to know from emergency radiologists. Emerg Radiol 2019. https://doi.org/10.1007/s10140-018-01662-z.

13. Zomorodi M. Nursing management: stroke. In: Lewis S, Heitkemper MM, Dirksen SR, et al, editors. Medical-surgical nursing: assessment and management of clinical problems. 10th edition. St Louis (MO): Mosby; 2016 (Chapter 58).

14. McLaughlin J. Brain, cranial, and maxillofacial trauma. In: Trauma nursing core course: an ENA course. Provider manual. 7th edition. Des Plaines (IL): Emergency Nurses Association; 2014. p. 105–22 (Chapter 9).

15. Nimmo G, Howie A, Grant I. Effects of mechanical ventilation on Cushing's triad. Crit Care 2009;13(1):77.

16. Hsiao P, Redley B, Hsiao Y, et al. Family needs of critically ill patients in the emergency department. Int J Emerg Med 2017;30:3–8.

17. Sather J, Rothenberg C, Finn EB, et al. Real-time surveys reveal important safety risks during interhospital care transitions for neurologic emergencies. Am J Med Qual 2018. https://doi.org/10.1177/1062860618785248.

18. Powers WJ, Rabinstein AA, Ackerson T, et al, American Heart Association Stroke Council. 2018 guidelines for the early management of patients with acute ischemic stroke: A guideline for healthcare professionals from the American Heart Association/American Stroke Association. Stroke 2018;49(3):e46–110.

19. Hemphill JC, Greenberg SM, Anderson CS, et al. Guidelines for the management of spontaneous intracerebral hemorrhage: a guideline for healthcare professionals from the American Heart Association/American Stroke Association. Stroke 2015;46(7):2032–60.

20. Connolly ES, Rabinstein AA, Carhuapoma JR, et al. Guidelines for the management of aneurysmal subarachnoid hemorrhage: a guideline for healthcare professionals from the American Heart Association/American Stroke Association. Stroke 2012;43(6):1711–37.

21. Brown R, Kumar A, McCullough L, et al. A survey of blood pressure parameters after aneurysmal subarachnoid hemorrhage. Int J Neurosci 2017;127:51–8.

22. Martino R, Foley N, Bhogal S, et al. Dysphagia after stroke: incidence, diagnosis, and pulmonary complications. Stroke 2005;36:2756–63.

23. Adams H, del Zoppo G, Alberts M, et al. Guidelines for the early management of adults with ischemic stroke: a guideline from the American Heart Association/American Stroke Association stroke council, clinical cardiology council, cardiovascular radiology and intervention council, and the atherosclerotic peripheral vascular disease and quality of care outcomes in research interdisciplinary working groups. Stroke 2007;38(5):1655–711.

24. Daniels S, Anderson J, Peterson N. Implementation of stroke dysphagia screening in the emergency department. Nurs Res Pract 2013. https://doi.org/10.1155/2013/304190.

25. Sivertsen J, Graverholt B, Espehaug B. Dysphagia screening after acute stroke: a quality improvement project using criteria-based clinical audit. BMC Nurs 2017; 16(27). https://doi.org/10.1186/s12912-017-0222-6.
26. Solet DJ, Norvell JM, Rutan GH, et al. Lost in translation: challenges and opportunities in physician-to- physician communication during patient hand-offs. Acad Med 2005;80:1094–9.
27. Hern H, Gallahue F, Burns B, et al. Handoff practices in emergency medicine: are we making progress? Acad Emerg Med 2016;23(2):197–201.
28. Lee S, Jordan J, Hern G, et al. Transition of care practices from emergency department to inpatient: survey data and development of algorithm. West J Emerg Med 2017;18(1):86–92.
29. Smith C, Britigan D, Lyden E, et al. Interunit handoffs from emergency department to inpatient care: a cross-sectional survey of physicians at a university medical center. J Hosp Med 2015;10(11):711–7.
30. Starmer AJ, Sectish TC, Simon DW, et al. Rates of medical errors and preventable adverse events among hospitalized children following implementation of a resident handoff bundle. JAMA 2013;310(21):2262–70.
31. Collins SA, Stein DM, Vawdrey DK, et al. Content overlap in nurse and physician handoff artifacts and the potential role of electronic health records: a systematic review. J Biomed Inform 2011;44(4):704–12.
32. McFetridge B, Gillespie M, Goode D, et al. An exploration of the process of critically ill patients between nursing staff from the emergency department and the intensive care unit. Nurs Crit Care 2007;12(6):261–9.

Handoff from Operating Room to Intensive Care Unit

Specific Pathways to Decrease Patient Adverse Events

Lori M. Rhudy, PhD, RN, CNRN, ACNS-BC

KEYWORDS

- Handover • Handoff surgery • Postoperative • Intensive care unit
- Transition of care • General surgery • Intensive care units

KEY POINTS

- Postoperative handoffs are critical to patient safety but there is a lack of consensus about what constitutes a good handoff.
- Successful handoff requires attendance and participation of all members of both care teams.
- Content of handoff report should be identified and vetted by all stakeholders with consideration of the unique contextual features of a setting or population.
- Standardized approaches to handoff can improve satisfaction with teamwork.
- Studies with larger sample size using rigorous methods are needed to understand the effect of operating room to intensive care unit handoff on adverse events.

INTRODUCTION

Handoffs are defined as "the transfer of professional responsibility and accountability for some or all aspects of care for a patient or group of patients to another person or professional group on a temporary or permanent basis."[1] Postoperative handoff is defined as the time during which the patient leaves the operating room (OR) and arrives at a postprocedural destination, such as the intensive care unit (ICU).[2] Handoff from the OR to the ICU involves a transfer of care between teams and is a higher-risk time for patient safety.[1] Handoffs from OR to ICU are complex, involving communication among multiple teams, including surgery, anesthesia, critical care, respiratory care, and nursing. Handoffs between the surgical and ICU teams involve many people

Disclosure: The author has no disclosures to report.
Department of Nursing, Division of Nursing Research, Mayo Clinic, 200 First Street Southwest, Rochester, MN 55905, USA
E-mail address: rhudy.lori@mayo.edu

at a single point of time, each with a specific focus for patient care, potentially increasing the risk of ineffective communication.[3,4] These transitions require the simultaneous physical relocation of both patient and equipment within time constraints.[2,5,6] The health care team must, at the same time, monitor the patient for potential complications and deliver or receive information about the patient, surgical procedure, and goals of care.[2] These complexities make unraveling the many factors that affect handoff quality challenging.

Numerous individual components that are required to transition patient care from the OR to ICU have been identified. Critical components of OR to ICU handoff include the efficient transition of monitors and other equipment, limiting discussions to those related to the patient, a face-to-face sharing of patient information and discussion of the plan of care between all providers involved, and limiting interruptions during the information handoff.[7]

Following the landmark Institute of Medicine reports[8,9] highlighting the impact of communication errors as factors leading to actual or potential medical errors, interest in strategies to improve communication between care providers has remained constant. In response, in 2006, the Joint Commission added 'Implement a standardized approach to "hand off" communications, including an opportunity to ask and respond to questions' to its National Patient Safety Goals; in 2010, that goal became a Joint Commission standard.[10,11] Since then, standardization efforts have resulted in the widespread development and implementation of handoff strategies, with varying degrees of success.[12] In 2011, the Accreditation Council for Graduate Medical Education instituted a requirement for resident training programs to provide formal education on handoffs and use a system to monitor quality of handoffs, further igniting the need for investigation into strategies to improve handoff of surgical patients.[13] Suggested strategies to improve handoffs and reduce medical errors include communication training, use of mnemonics to guide handoffs, required participation of all team members, and the use of written or computerized guides or checklists.[14]

Strength and Quality of the Evidence

Systematic reviews and meta-analysis are most often at the top of evidence hierarchies used to aid in classifying evidence.[15] Handoff from OR to ICU has garnered enough interest and examination to be the focus of several high-quality systematic reviews[2,12,16,17]; however, none of the systematic reviews were able to generate strong recommendations for practice. In addition, systematic reviews of a variety of interclinician handoffs (eg, postoperative, change of shift) identify similar interventions to improve handoff communication, which include standardized processes, training and education, changes to the physical environment, use of technology, and explicit transfer of responsibility.[18,19] Segall and colleagues[17] reviewed 34 articles that specifically addressed postoperative handoff to ICU or postanesthesia care unit (PACU). Despite their appraisal that the quality of evidence was variable and strong evidence was lacking, they identified 5 interventions that were broadly supported:

- Standardized processes using checklists and protocols
- Completion of urgent tasks before information transfer
- Allow only patient-specific discussion during handoff
- Require that all relevant team members be present for handoff
- Provide training in team skills and communication

Segall and colleagues[17] listed 74 elements and Mukhopadhyay and colleagues[20] identified 49 elements from the existing literature as necessary for an effective OR to ICU handoff. This finding points to the multifaceted and contextually dependent nature of handoffs. From both research and practice perspectives, addressing a large number of factors for implementation and then teasing out which elements might improve outcomes associated with OR to ICU handoff is a daunting task.

Only 1 study of OR to ICU handoff in neurosurgical patients[6] is available. This article focuses on the factors prominent in the literature that may inform practice in neurosurgical settings. These factors include prehandoff activities, inclusion of relevant team members, contextual factors, structured handoff tools, homogenous populations, novel interventions, outcome measures, and implications for future research.

Prehandoff Activities

Because transfer of a patient from OR to ICU requires not only verbal handoff but also the physical transfer of equipment such as monitors, tubes, and lines, preparation by the receiving ICU team is a necessary component to make sure the environment is appropriate and to ensure the team members are available for handoff. A variety of strategies have been proposed to initiate handoff before the arrival of the patient in the ICU. Some protocols include a call from OR to ICU at key points in the surgical procedure, such as after induction or incision, at closing, and/or just before leaving the OR (often referred to as rolling),[20–26] to ready the receiving team for the patient's arrival. Other interventions defined specific time frames for pretransfer communication; for example, 30 minutes before anticipated transfer.[22,27] In many cases, a combination of these alerts were used, such as a call after induction and again just before transfer. For example, Mukhopadhyay and colleagues[20] instituted a pretransfer call to the ICU nurse with information about the procedure, lines, drips, and ventilator status so that the receiving nurse could physically prepare for the patient's arrival.[20] Nursing staff then contacted the ICU provider as soon as the patient arrived in the unit. One protocol used the electronic health record (EHR) to provide advance warning at induction and near the end of the procedure.[25] Another used a printout of a report generated from OR data in the EHR to provide advance information about the patient,[24] whereas another used completion of a written SBAR (situation, background, assessment, recommendation) form.[26] Despite the inclusion of prehandoff activities in nearly all published OR to ICU handoff protocols, whether these activities influence the handoff process or outcomes has received little attention.[28]

Relevant Team Members

Patient care in the OR as well as in the ICU is delivered by a multidisciplinary team that includes surgeons, anesthesiologists, certified registered nurse anesthetists, registered nurses (RNs), nurse practitioners, physician assistants, respiratory therapists, and others. The transfer of critically ill patients from the OR to the surgical ICU requires not only the verbal handoff of information but also a physical handoff of patient and equipment between 2 distinct treatment teams, leaving multiple points for communication breakdown and information loss to occur.[20] Efforts to standardize OR to ICU handoff have found that requiring all relevant team members be present and actively engaged in the handoff is critical.[6,20,21,24] Competing priorities such as surgeon need to return to the OR for another procedure, patient instability, and other patient care needs in the ICU are factors that may result in team members being absent from or leaving early in the handoff.[23,29] Despite a highly prescriptive protocol, including even the order in which equipment should be transferred, Krimminger and colleagues[24] observed that implementation of a new handoff process did not result in significant change in separation of handoff report from patient activity, further highlighting the multitasking that occurs during OR to ICU handoffs.

Team work has been identified as both a key factor in the handoff process and a key outcome of handoff improvement initiatives.[4,30] Preimplementation evaluation has shown that identification of care team members occurs in only a small number of handoffs.[20,21] Reports show that in preintervention phases it was common for handoff to occur without nursing or respiratory therapy,[21] without ICU physician providers,[5,20] or without a member of the surgical team[20,31] present. One common step in OR to ICU handoff intervention studies is to include a time-out to ensure all team members were present and ready to receive report.[21,26]

Introduction of each caregiver present is also a common feature of standardized handoff processes that allows the team to ensure all necessary parties are present. Following teamwork best practices, identification of a single provider from the team to provide leadership in directing the handoff or prompting for missing information may improve outcomes further.[20] Which care team member is the leader and how this is implemented varies across settings. One setting implemented a time-out in which the surgical resident began the handoff process[21]; in others, the receiving ICU RN[23] or anesthesia provider[20,26,32] initiated the handoff.

Structured Handoff Tools

The development of standardized tools to direct the content and process of handoff has been widely hypothesized as a strategy to improve handoff. Standardized tools are thought to reduce the loss of information and improve quality of the handoff, potentially resulting in fewer postoperative complications in the first 24 postoperative hours.[1] In an integrated review, all 7 interventional studies showed reduced information omissions and improvement in amount of critical information transferred during handoff after implementation of a structured handoff tool.[3] Information included in structured handoff tools was generally decided by key stakeholders, from previous research, or by identifying areas prone to high consequence error.[2,3] This information was then arranged into checklists or scripts used to guide and/or evaluate handoff. Checklists are often organized by categories such as demographics, patient history, anesthesia information, surgical information, and postoperative information.[3] Some guides focus on tasks such as timing and content of prehandoff calls, how the handoff is initiated, or the order in which information is provided. There is wide variability on what and how much information is considered critical elements of checklists.

Contextual Factors in Implementation

Studies that design, implement, and test evidence-based approaches to standardized handoff from OR to ICU have shown the need for attention to context and key stakeholder buy-in.[3,23] An integrated review concluded that flexibility in structured handoff tool development is warranted because rigid standardization processes and tools that do not allow for contextual needs perform poorly.[3] Similarly, participants in the Handoffs and Transitions in Critical Care (HATRICC) study voiced concern that too much focus on completion of checklists or tools to guide handoff could be distractors to the actual handoff, which could lead to important information not considered in the checklist being overlooked.[23] Lane-Fall and colleagues[23] addressed this barrier by implementing a template that did not have specific rules about who would complete it or specific details that must be included, but instead included suggestions for information that might be needed by the receiver, making it more flexible for the mixed surgical procedures in the study.

One goal of the handoff process, in addition to a safe and efficient transition of care from the OR to the ICU, is for the different professionals on the care team to have a shared understanding of patient status, expected trajectory, and clinical priorities.[4,33]

Focus groups with PACU nurses, anesthesiologists, and nurse anesthetists showed differing perspectives about postoperative handoffs in each group.[4] Key findings included different temporal perspectives on the handoff (past, present, or future focus), uncertainty about whether all of the information needed was actually transferred from one team to another, different views on when and whether transfer of responsibility occurred, and desire to ensure high-quality handoff by focusing on things out of the normal course of events.

Homogenous Populations

Interpretation and implementation of findings from studies of handoff from OR to ICU is challenging in part because of the homogenous populations in which this aspect of care has been studied. Handoff of both pediatric and adult cardiac surgery patients are the most studied OR to ICU handoffs, probably because of the large number of cases compared with other specialties. The overall number of surgical and anesthesia providers involved in care in mixed-population ICUs in most institutions dwarfs the usual number of pediatric surgeons and cardiac anesthesia providers, making the logistics of education, training, and adherence more challenging in multispecialty settings.[21] In addition, the anticipated complications are likely more predictable within this population, making identification of standardized patient outcomes easier. For example, Hall and colleagues[25] conducted a preintervention-postintervention study of 1127 postoperative cardiac surgery admissions using a critical care complication registry database containing data about all patients in this setting to examine complications. A list of 26 possible complications was identified with preventable and/or serious complications derived from the original list by consensus of intensivists.[25] Preventable complications were those in which it was "believed that transfer of operative or preoperative information at the time of handover could significantly decrease the probability of the complication."[25(p478)] Serious complications were those associated with new organ failure. Results showed that preventable complications declined from 29 to 11 ($P = .023$) before and after the intervention with no statistical difference in serious complications. The exchange of critical patient information, including the patient's medical history, the surgical procedure performed, and any events of concern that occurred during the surgery, are key elements of the handoff from OR to ICU care teams.[24] It is possible that the vital information for cardiovascular patients is more easily standardized than for other specialty populations. More recently, research on interventions to improve handoff in other surgical populations has been undertaken, including multispecialty pediatric ICU,[21] mixed surgical ICU,[20,23] all ICUs in an organization,[24,34] and neurosurgery patients in China.[6]

The bulk of evidence on handoff from OR to ICU involves implementation and evaluation in a single ICU. However, more recently efforts to advance this work to other specialties and across multiple units are emerging. For example, Lane-Fall and colleagues[23] in the HATRICC study developed an OR to ICU handoff process for use in 2 mixed surgical ICUs. In a randomized controlled trial of 121 handoffs in many surgical specialties (abdominal, gynecology, urology, ear/nose/throat, oral/maxillofacial, orthopedic/trauma, neurosurgery, spine, neuroradiology, and vascular surgeries), handoffs were randomized to checklist-guided handoff or not followed by audio recording of the handoff.[34] The handoffs were analyzed via assessment of the percentage of items handed over from the caregiving anesthesiologist (resident) to the ICU physician and ICU nurse that were declared as important to be handed over by the supervising anesthesiologist. An average of 17 items per patient were determined as red items (must be handed over); an average of 3 yellow (should be handed over) items per patient were identified. The intervention group using the checklist showed a statistically significant difference in number of red items handed off but no significant difference was found in handoff of yellow items.

Novel Interventions in Handoff Research

In general, descriptions of handoff from OR to ICU follow a predictable format with only minor modifications based on the unique context. The most commonly used intervention to address handoff communication from OR to ICU is implementation of checklist, template, and/or script to guide the transfer of information. However, a few investigators have identified different strategies to address the problem. Simulation was used to aid development of a redesigned OR to ICU handoff process.[30] Catchpole and colleagues[32] used the analogy of pit stops similar to those used by Formula 1 racing teams to define handoff steps. Using this model, they described handoff in 4 phases and identified the key activities and information at each phase. A key factor addressed in their process was designation of a leader for the handoff process; however, findings did not necessarily show that the new process improved teamwork. Although it is often cited, no replication has been reported.

Lane-Fall and colleagues[23] used dance as an analogy to describe a choreographed handoff process developed with consideration of the preexisting work-flow patterns of clinician movement. The resulting process involved a series of steps, each with defined actors and content. For example, the surgeon reports first, then the anesthesiologist with templates used to guide the information content. Kimminger and colleagues[24] developed a similar process, as described in other studies, but in addition emphasized the need for no interruptions during handoff. Riley and colleagues[33] identified 1 outcome of OR to ICU handoff, being formation of a shared mental model of patient status and clinical priorities. Their intervention included a 1 to 5 repeat-back tool used in handoff. The tool included I know: what is wrong; what to do; what to worry about; when to escalate; and what you see.

Mnemonics to guide handoff are gaining increasing popularity. The mnemonic I-PASS (illness severity, patient summary, action list, situation awareness and contingency plans, and synthesis by receiver) was developed as a guide for oral and written handoffs between resident physicians.[29] Participation in the I-PASS curriculum improved perceived interclinician communication, preparedness, and work flow and patient safety between residents, fellows, attending physicians, and advance practice clinicians, but objective outcome data showed no improvement in ICU length of stay, ventilator days, or reintubation rates.[35] A REDCap database was used to house a handoff tool based on the I-PASS mnemonic.[29] Handoffs from OR to ICU or stepdown unit were entered into the database; residents received a prompt to make a phone call for watchers or face-to-face handoff if a patient was unstable. After intervention, improvements in handoff compliance, documented postoperative checks, and decreased communication errors and time needed to create action lists for the shift were observed, although the study included all handoffs, not only those from OR to ICU. The I-PASS structure for handoff has been primarily implemented and tested in physician to physician handoff. Whether it has broader applicability to handoffs between teams such as OR to ICU needs to be investigated.

Another mnemonic, PETS, includes prehandoff, equipment and monitor, time-out, and sign out.[26] Prehandoff includes preparation of the SBAR document; call to the receiving unit; and preparation of monitors, drains, and drips for transfer. This prehandoff is followed by the handoff of equipment and monitor, time-out in which the SBAR form is discussed, and then the sign-out phase in which the surgeon, anesthetist, and receiving physician agree on the plan for the patient, identify anticipated problems, and anticipated course of recovery. Nurses' rating of handoff information as sufficient improved from 32% to 96%.[26]

Evaluation of video recordings to determine tempo and quality of handoffs was used to test the hypothesis that OR to ICU handoff quality (engagement, teamwork, and report delivery skills) would be lower on nights and weekends because of provider fatigue and decreased schedule predictability.[5] Instead, findings suggested that handoff performance on nights and weekends was similar, and in some cases better than on weekdays.[5] These investigators suggested that lighter operative caseloads led to providers being less rushed or distracted, which enabled them to be more engaged in the handoff, and that the study was limited by the very small number of handoffs (16) observed in each group. Similarly, observation of handoffs to compare handoff quality on nights/weekends compared with weekdays showed that OR to ICU handoff quality was similar or superior on off hours and that quality was better in the unit with higher patient volumes.[36] The investigators surmise that more senior surgery and anesthesia residents are involved in care during the off hours, making them more knowledgeable about the entire surgical procedure and therefore better able to deliver more relevant information.

Outcome Measures

Adverse outcomes caused by handoff failures are typically the result of a cascade of events that are difficult to attribute solely to handoff mistakes, which makes the estimation and investigation of handoff quality and related errors difficult,[18] in part because no universal definition or standard tool to assess handoff quality exists.[2,12] Systematic reviews found that most studies used handoff activity–related outcome measures, including accuracy of information as measured by number of errors or adherence to a checklist, duration of handoff, number of patients handed off, interruptions, care quality, frequency of tool use, handoff efficiency, and length of shift report.[2,12] Yang and Zhang[6] in addition to evaluating handoff process outcomes also measured immediate postoperative patient outcomes of ventilator weaning within the first 6 hours after ICU admission and duration of mechanical ventilation. The sample of 102 patients was adequately powered to meet the study aims and showed significant results for decrease in ventilation duration from 5.1 to 3.3 hours, and 6-hour weaning increased from 70% to 82% but was not statistically significant. A systematic review of interventions used in intrahospital transfers found that, in the 15 studies included, 82 discrete outcome measures were evaluated.[18] Secondary outcomes reflecting handoff attendance, antibiotic delays, time to analgesia doses, and postoperative pain scores have been evaluated.[21]

None of the published reports found a significant change in the amount of time required for OR to ICU handoff. Improved perception of teamwork and quality of handoff is an almost universally reported outcome of handoff improvement efforts. Abraham and colleagues[12] suggest that the use of handoff-related measures provides only narrow or local metrics that are not easily linked to patient outcome data on patient safety and continuity. Proposed patient outcomes more reflective of handoff quality include procedural or treatment delays, adverse patient events, rehospitalization rates, number of returns to the OR, and length of stay in the ICU.[27]

Few studies examine sustainability of handoff improvement initiatives beyond the first few months to year after implementation. Chenault and colleagues[37] evaluated outcomes 5 years after initial implementation and found that technical errors and verbal information omissions were significantly reduced compared with preintervention and immediate postintervention time frames. Riley and colleagues[33] evaluated their intervention at 8 weeks, 1 year, 3 years, and 4 years and found that, at 4 years, compliance with the process remained greater than 75%, and additional improvements in compliance in most measures occurred between 8 weeks and 4 years. Surveys administered 3 years after implementation showed significantly higher satisfaction with the new handoff process.[30]

Neurosurgery Transitions

There is little evidence specifically focused on critical elements of transitions from neurosurgery OR to ICU. However, information considered essential in general neurosurgery handoffs can inform key information needed for neurosurgery OR to ICU handoff. In one study, the mnemonic SAAFE (sick patients, after surgery, admissions, follow closely, and essential run through) was used to facilitate shift sign-out in neurosurgery.[38] Specific elements of SAAFE relevant to the OR to ICU handoff include admitting diagnosis, past medical history, neurologic status, current treatment plan and rationale, and potential therapeutic plan in the event of clinical decline. Postoperative transfer and management in an ICU allows for rapid detection of neurologic, hemodynamic, metabolic, or respiratory complication associated with intracranial surgery.[39] In a study of 167 patients with craniotomy for intracranial tumor, 45% experienced a postoperative complication and, of those, 85% were in the first 2 hours after surgery, and postoperative nausea and vomiting was the most common complication.[39] Thus, as shown in other surgical populations, a description of the surgical course and any complications during surgery should be communicated to the receiving team with an identified action plan. In one protocol designed to improve handoff of neurosurgery patients to ICU, recommended content included surgical information such as procedure, estimated blood loss, and surgical site information and plans care such as fluid management, pain management and sedation, ventilator weaning and extubation, and feeding.[6]

As described for other specialty populations, transfer of equipment and monitors, such as intracranial pressure monitors and external ventricular drains, is a necessary part of the OR to ICU transfer of neurosurgical patients and should be considered in the pretransfer communication to ensure the environment is ready. In addition, specific parameters for care, such as management of external ventricular drainage, electroencephalogram monitoring, and timing of radiologic assessments, are important to the critical care team assuming care.

Team training should be considered a key part of any strategy designed to improve handoffs from neurosurgical suite to ICU. In one study of 449 neurosurgical residents, 63% reported no formal instruction in handoffs.[40] Using a standardized process to improve neurosurgery to ICU handoff in mainland China, Yang and Zhang[6] showed improvements in teamwork scores. Reporting of surgical information increased from 42% to 83%, whereas anesthesia information increased from 75% to 93% with the addition of a checklist and required the presence of all team members.

Implications for Future Research

Although randomized controlled trials are preferred because of their scientific rigor, it is often challenging to conduct these in clinical settings because of a variety of factors: challenges of incorporating a new intervention without disrupting the existing workflow, recruiting a random sample of clinicians, lack of universally accepted outcome and evaluation measures for handoffs, and difficulty in linking to patient-related data for evaluation. The need to adjust interventions to address the unique patient and setting contexts further adds to the difficulty. Given that randomized controlled trials may not be feasible in most settings for evaluating handoff outcomes, alternatives

> **Box 1**
> **Research opportunities**
>
> - Identify and test patient-centered outcomes related to handoff
> - Examine the influence of prehandoff activities in relation to the overall handoff process and outcomes
> - Describe strategies to sustain handoff improvements over time
> - Develop taxonomies for handoff to allow better discussion and comparison across studies
> - Investigate outcomes in highly defined compared with more flexible handoff strategies
> - Test and translate findings from existing studies to broader populations

need to be explored.[12] Investigators in studies of OR to ICU handoffs have called for the use of larger sample sizes, mixed populations, and more transparency in intervention development processes and tools so that they can be reused and/or replicated. Scientific work is needed to achieve the goals listed in **Box 1.**

DISCUSSION

Because communication failures have been shown as key factors in errors, The Joint Commission emphasized the need for standardized handoff. However, what this looks like in practice is not defined. When it comes to the transition of patients from the OR team to the ICU team, research studies and quality-improvement initiatives to standardize handoff have included the use of scripts, checklists, and early warning of transfer followed by observation and survey to measure the impact of these interventions. Comparison across studies is challenging because strategies and outcomes are not defined or measured consistently. Most of the work in this area is not powered adequately to determine the effect on patient outcomes. So, although provider satisfaction is improved, whether these strategies meet their intended goal to improve patient safety is difficult to evaluate.

Future studies should focus on the multiple functions of handoff (information transfer, shared understanding, and teamwork) rather than only on standardized information transfer.[2] The research is limited in that almost all is focused on cardiovascular (CV) surgery contexts, both pediatric and adult. Whether the standardized content developed for CV surgery will be effective in other populations is unclear and warrants further examination. In addition, the ability to generalize is limited, with many of the reports being quality-improvement initiatives designed to improve practice in a particular setting. Developing multifaceted care interventions that are sensitive to organizational context and clinician work flow is a key principle in the human factors approach required to address handoff as a patient safety initiative.[23,37]

REFERENCES

1. Agarwal HS, Saville BR, Slayton JM, et al. Standardized postoperative handover process improves outcomes in the intensive care unit: a model for operational sustainability and improved team performance*. Crit Care Med 2012;40(7): 2109–15.
2. Moller TP, Madsen MD, Fuhrmann L, et al. Postoperative handover: characteristics and considerations on improvement: a systematic review. Eur J Anaesthesiol 2013;30(5):229–42.

3. Gardiner TM, Marshall AP, Gillespie BM. Clinical handover of the critically ill postoperative patient: an integrative review. Aust Crit Care 2015;28(4):226–34.

4. Randmaa M, Engstrom M, Swenne CL, et al. The postoperative handover: a focus group interview study with nurse anaesthetists, anaesthesiologists and PACU nurses. BMJ Open 2017;7(8):e015038.

5. Barry ME, Hochman BR, Lane-Fall MB, et al. Leveraging telemedicine infrastructure to monitor quality of operating room to intensive care unit handoffs. Acad Med 2017;92(7):1035–42.

6. Yang JG, Zhang J. Improving the postoperative handover process in the intensive care unit of a tertiary teaching hospital. J Clin Nurs 2016;25(7–8):1062–72.

7. Joy BF, Elliott E, Hardy C, et al. Standardized multidisciplinary protocol improves handover of cardiac surgery patients to the intensive care unit. Pediatr Crit Care Med 2011;12(3):304–8.

8. Institute of Medicine Committee on Quality of Health Care in A. Crossing the quality Chasm: a new health system for the 21st century. In: Crossing the quality Chasm: a new health system for the 21st century. Washington, DC: National Academies Press (US) Copyright 2001 by the National Academy of Sciences. All rights reserved; 2001.

9. Institute of Medicine. Crossing the quality chasm: a new health system for the 21st century. Washington, DC: The National Academies Press; 2001.

10. Cohen MD, Hilligoss PB. The published literature on handoffs in hospitals: deficiencies identified in an extensive review. Qual Saf Health Care 2010;19(6):493.

11. The Joint Commission. Inadequate hand-off communication. Sentinel Event Alert 2017;(58):1–6.

12. Abraham J, Kannampallil T, Patel VL. A systematic review of the literature on the evaluation of handoff tools: implications for research and practice. J Am Med Inform Assoc 2014;21(1):154–62.

13. Nasca TJ, Day SH, Amis ES. The new recommendations on duty hours from the ACGME task force. N Engl J Med 2010;363(2):e3.

14. Starmer AJ, Sectish TC, Simon DW, et al. Rates of medical errors and preventable adverse events among hospitalized children following implementation of a resident handoff bundle. JAMA 2013;310(21):2262–70.

15. Melnyk BM, Fineout-Overholt E. Evidence-based practice in nursing & healthcare. 2nd edition. Lippincott, Williams & Wilkins; 2011.

16. Pucher PH, Johnston MJ, Aggarwal R, et al. Effectiveness of interventions to improve patient handover in surgery: a systematic review. Surgery 2015;158(1):85–95.

17. Segall N, Bonifacio AS, Schroeder RA, et al. Can we make postoperative patient handovers safer? A systematic review of the literature. Anesth Analg 2012;115(1):102–15.

18. Robertson ER, Morgan L, Bird S, et al. Interventions employed to improve intrahospital handover: a systematic review. BMJ Qual Saf 2014;23(7):600–7.

19. Davis J, Roach C, Elliott C, et al. Feedback and assessment tools for handoffs: a systematic review. J Grad Med Educ 2017;9(1):18–32.

20. Mukhopadhyay D, Wiggins-Dohlvik KC, MrDutt MM, et al. Implementation of a standardized handoff protocol for post-operative admissions to the surgical intensive care unit. Am J Surg 2018;215(1):28–36.

21. Breuer RK, Taicher B, Turner DA, et al. Standardizing postoperative PICU handovers improves handover metrics and patient outcomes. Pediatr Crit Care Med 2015;16(3):256–63.

22. Dixon JL, Stagg HW, Wehbe-Janek H, et al. A standard handoff improves cardiac surgical patient transfer: operating room to intensive care unit. J Healthc Qual 2015;37(1):22–32.
23. Lane-Fall M, Pascual JL, Massa S, et al. Developing a standard handoff process for operating room–to-ICU transitions: multidisciplinary clinician perspectives from the handoffs and transitions in critical care (HATRICC) study. Jt Comm J Qual Patient Saf 2018;44:514–25.
24. Krimminger D, Sona C, Thomas-Horton E, et al. A Multidisciplinary QI initiative to improve OR-ICU handovers. Am J Nurs 2018;118(2):48–59.
25. Hall M, Robertson J, Merkel M, et al. A structured transfer of care process reduces perioperative complications in cardiac surgery patients. Anesth Analg 2017;125(2):477–82.
26. Fabila TS, Hee HI, Sultana R, et al. Improving postoperative handover from anaesthetists to non-anaesthetists in a children's intensive care unit: the receiver's perception. Singapore Med J 2016;57(5):242–53.
27. Van Der Walt JJN, Scholl AT, Joubert IA, et al. Implementation of a postoperative handoff protocol. South Afr J Anaesth Analg 2016;22(6):33–7.
28. Haque SN, Osterlund CS, Fagan LM. What's ideal? A case study exploring handoff routines in practice. J Biomed Inform 2017;65:159–67.
29. Clarke CN, Patel SH, Day RW, et al. Implementation of a standardized electronic tool improves compliance, accuracy, and efficiency of trainee-to-trainee patient care handoffs after complex general surgical oncology procedures. Surgery 2017;161(3):869–75.
30. Segall N, Bonifacio AS, Barbeito A, et al. Operating room-to-ICU patient handovers: a multidisciplinary human-centered design approach. Jt Comm J Qual Patient Saf 2016;42(9):400–14.
31. Judging handoffs: video study validates tool. Hosp Peer Rev 2014;39(9):104–5.
32. Catchpole KR, De Leval MR, McEwan A, et al. Patient handover from surgery to intensive care: using formula 1 pit-stop and aviation models to improve safety and quality. Paediatr Anaesth 2007;17(5):470–8.
33. Riley CM, Merritt AD, Mize JM, et al. Assuring sustainable gains in interdisciplinary performance improvement: creating a shared mental model during operating room to cardiac ICU handoff. Pediatr Crit Care Med 2017;18(9):863–8.
34. Salzwedel C, Mai V, Punke MA, et al. The effect of a checklist on the quality of patient handover from the operating room to the intensive care unit: a randomized controlled trial. J Crit Care 2016;32:170–4.
35. Parent B, LaGrone LN, Albirair MT, et al. Effect of standardized handoff curriculum on improved clinician preparedness in the intensive care unit a stepped-wedge cluster randomized clinical trial. JAMA Surg 2018;153(5):464–70.
36. Hochman BR, Barry ME, Lane-Fall MB, et al. Handoffs in the intensive care unit. Am J Med Qual 2017;32(2):186–93.
37. Chenault K, Moga MA, Shin M, et al. Sustainability of protocolized handover of pediatric cardiac surgery patients to the intensive care unit. Paediatr Anaesth 2016;26(5):488–94.
38. Falla A, Ibrahim GM, Bernstein M. The SAAFE neurosurgical sign-out. World Neurosurg 2014;81(3–4):e21–3.
39. Lonjaret L, Guyonnet M, Berard E, et al. Postoperative complications after craniotomy for brain tumor surgery. Anaesth Crit Care Pain Med 2017;36(4):213–8.
40. Babu MA, Nahed BV, Heary RF. Investigating the scope of resident patient care handoffs within neurosurgery. PLoS One 2012;7(7):e41810.

Transitions of Care for Patients with Neurologic Diagnoses Transition from the Intensive Care Unit to the Floor

Molly McNett, PhD, RN, CNRN, FNCS[a],[*],
Diane McLaughlin, DNP, APRN-CNP, AGACNP-BC[b]

KEYWORDS

- Transition of care • Neurocritical care • Patient transfer • Neurology • Neurosurgery

KEY POINTS

- Successful transition from the intensive care unit to the acute care unit or nursing floor promotes recovery and reduces risk of adverse events among patients with acute neurologic injury.
- Deescalation of frequent and invasive monitoring modalities is a crucial component for successful transition to acute care units.
- Timely and accurate handoff techniques among interdisciplinary teams promote successful transitions by limiting errors and streamlining discharge processes to promote recovery.
- Knowledge of risk factors for readmission to the intensive care unit is important to mitigate risk and aid in recognition of symptoms to facilitate early interventions.

INTRODUCTION

Transition of care from the intensive care unit (ICU) to an acute care unit includes evaluation of a variety of factors to assess readiness for ICU discharge and to ensure continuity of care and patient safety. Ongoing communication with the clinical team, patients, and family members is essential to optimize transitions from a higher level of care and to continue the trajectory of discharge planning and patient recovery. Specific considerations regarding clinical components, patient status, and family preferences must factor into transition decisions. Transition begins with the deescalation of ICU monitoring, which includes neurologic assessments, invasive monitoring

[a] Implementation Science Core, The Helene Fuld Health Trust National Institute for EBP, College of Nursing, 760 Kinnear Road, Columbus, OH 43212, USA; [b] Neurocritical Care and Neurosurgery, The MetroHealth System, Case Western Reserve University, MetroHealth Medical Center, 2500 MetroHealth Drive, Attn: Nursing Business Office, Cleveland, OH 44109, USA
* Corresponding author.
E-mail address: mcnett.21@osu.edu

Nurs Clin N Am 54 (2019) 347–355
https://doi.org/10.1016/j.cnur.2019.04.005
0029-6465/19/© 2019 Elsevier Inc. All rights reserved.

technologies, electrolyte maintenance, electroencephalogram (EEG) monitoring, and hemodynamic parameters. A primary tenet of the transition process is effective hand-off communication between ICU and acute care unit interdisciplinary teams. Initial management of care in acute care settings focuses on agitation management, assessing readiness for discharge, and preventing complications leading to ICU readmission.

Deescalation of Intensive Care Monitoring

Perhaps the most important transition decision centers on assessment of readiness for transfer from ICU settings to acute care units. Clinical components often drive these assessments. In critically ill patients with neurologic injury, clinical components include frequency of neurologic assessments, weaning from intracranial pressure (ICP monitoring and external ventricular drain drainage), evaluating the need for EEG monitoring, stability of laboratory values, and hemodynamic monitoring. The management of a patient after acute neurologic injury exists on a continuum from emergency to critical to general medical care. Although few recommendations exist to guide the deescalation of critical care management of neurologic issues, the neurologic assessments section highlights key considerations when preparing the transition of a patient with neurologic injury from the ICU to the acute care unit, and centers primarily on deescalation strategies to optimize outcomes and decrease the risk of ICU readmission.

Neurologic assessments

Serial neurologic assessments are a cornerstone of care monitoring in ICU settings. Often the need for serial, close surveillance of neurologic status is a priority indication for admission to a neurocritical ICU. Many acute care units may not have resources to provide close monitoring and frequent serial neurologic examinations. Hence, admission to ICU settings is warranted to provide this level of monitoring until the patient status stabilizes. Historically, serial neurologic examinations occur every hour; however, many neurointensivists have recently begun to balance risk of missing neurologic deterioration against risk of sleep deprivation among critically ill patients after neurologic injury.[1] The risk for neurologic deterioration often depends on the neurologic condition being managed, because common timeframes for acute deterioration may vary among patient populations. The need for frequent, serial neurologic assessments often mandates continued ICU care; as the frequency of these neurologic assessments decreases, transition to acute care units may be considered.

Some neurologic injuries have well-established monitoring parameters for serial neurologic assessments that mandate ICU care for set periods before transition to acute care settings. Patients experiencing ischemic stroke who receive intravenous alteplase must be monitored every 15 minutes for 4 hours, then every 30 minutes for 4 hours, then every hour for the duration of 24 hours.[2] This frequent monitoring occurs to observe for signs of hemorrhagic conversion, which occurs in up to 27% of patients during 2 to 6 hours.[3] Similarly, young patients with ischemic stroke, owing to large vessel occlusion, are often monitored every hour if deemed to be at high risk for cerebral edema necessitating emergent decompressive hemicraniectomy. Although it may be unusual for these patients to acutely deteriorate, serial neurologic assessments are required to detect critical changes in neurologic status and ongoing ICU care is warranted. The stability of a neurologic assessment and decreased requirements for frequent neurologic assessments are often a first step toward preparing for transition from the ICU setting to an acute care floor setting. Astute documentation in the electronic medical record of serial neurologic assessments while in the ICU can serve as a critical reference for nurses on the floor, particularly if the patient experiences a neurologic change after ICU discharge. Documentation of prior neurologic assessments, as well as clear communication at the time of transfer, can provide floor nurses with knowledge of subtle nuances of a patient's neurologic status over time.

Among patients with intracranial hemorrhage, hourly neurologic assessments are required until there is neurologic and radiographic stability, which often depends on the size of the hemorrhage. Typically, the first 48 hours after the initial hemorrhage are associated with the highest risk of deterioration and ongoing ICU monitoring is required.[4] Similarly, patients with aneurysmal subarachnoid hemorrhage are at high risk for aneurysm rerupture, and require hourly neurologic examinations both before and after aneurysm securement.[5] The ongoing risk for vasospasm remains high for up to 21 days, and the frequency of neurologic assessments may be deescalated and reescalated based on patient symptoms.[5] Regardless of the etiology of the neurologic injury, transition to an acute care floor is highly dependent on the risk for acute neurologic decompensation and predicated on the frequency of neurologic assessments. As risk decreases and neurologic examinations stabilize, the frequency of these assessments may be decreased, and considerations for transfer to acute care units may be considered if other parameters have stabilized.

Intracranial pressure monitoring

Monitoring of ICP is another key factor impacting transition from ICU settings to acute care units. The invasive nature of this monitoring mandates ICU care, and transfer to an acute care settings cannot be considered until ICP values have stabilized and invasive monitoring is no longer warranted. The measurement of ICP can be essential to the survival of patients with an acute brain injury.[6] Two common methods of measuring include the placement of an intraparenchymal bolt, or an extraventricular drain, both of which can prevent transfer to floor settings.

The ability to wean patients from this type of ICP monitoring is a vital consideration in deescalation of ICU care to assess readiness for transfer to acute care units. Weaning from ICP monitoring should be considered after stable neurologic improvement, resolution of elevated ICP, or resolution of hydrocephalus. In some patients, these goals will never be reached and it is the responsibility of the treatment team to determine the risks and benefits of continued ICP monitoring or cerebral spinal fluid diversion. Some patients may demonstrate need for a ventriculoperitoneal shunt if external ventricular drain weaning is unsuccessful. One retrospective study demonstrated a need for ventriculoperitoneal shunt after hydrocephalus after subarachnoid hemorrhage in 60% of patients.[7] If the ICP parameters remain stable, monitoring may be withdrawn and ventriculoperitoneal shunt placement may be performed as indicated as part of the overall deescalation of care in preparation for transfer to the floor.

Continuous electroencephalogram

Continuous EEG (cEEG) monitoring is another commonly used device in ICUs after neurologic injury, and should be effectively deescalated before transition to acute care units. Continuous EEG monitoring is typically used for the diagnosis of seizure tendency, evaluation for nocturnal seizures, and to determine the type and location of the seizure focus. The most common indication for EEG monitoring in the ICU is to evaluate for the presence of nonconvulsive status epilepticus as a cause of altered mental status or coma.[7] Oftentimes this is done with a routine 20- to 30-minute EEG, although the success of diagnosing intermittent nonconvulsive seizure activity does increase over duration of monitoring, with most being identified within 24 to 48 hours.[8] If status epilepticus is diagnosed, cEEG is necessary to evaluate response to treatment, because motor activity often ceases before status epilepticus.[9]

When seizures are adequately controlled for 12 to 24 hours, cEEG is maintained as medications, such as diprivan, ketamine, or midazolam, are weaned while observing for recurrence of seizures or status. There is no clear guideline regarding whether some seizure activity should be tolerated while these medications are weaned off or if the absence of seizures entirely should be the goal of weaning.[9] Most patients are maintained on antiepileptic drugs throughout the acute care unit stay, with weaning of these medications not attempted during the acute phase of brain injury.

Continuous EEG monitoring usually can be safely discontinued in patients without seizures within 48 hours from time of last seizure in patients with status epilepticus, or among patients being evaluated for possible status epilepticus. The health care team should maintain seizures as a possible diagnosis among patients who do not return to baseline neurologic status regardless of the period of cEEG monitoring, because the absence of seizure activity on the EEG does not rule out previous or future seizures. It is critical that this information be effectively communicated among provider teams as patients transition to acute care settings to ensure continuity of monitoring and clinical care. Communication should include documentation in the electronic medical record and verbally during the handoff and transferring process.

Laboratory Monitoring

Sodium imbalances are often the most common electrolyte abnormality after neurologic injury. Ongoing ICU care includes the stabilization of these laboratory values before transfer to acute care units. During ICU care, induced hypernatremia may be initiated by administering hypertonic saline to move interstitial and intracellular fluid into the intravascular space, and thus decrease cerebral edema temporarily; however, avoidance of hyponatremia remains the ultimate goal.[10–12] Not only must cerebral edema be managed before transfer to acute care units, but stabilization of sodium levels must also occur. Hyponatremia may be common after neurologic injury, and has been associated with neurologic decline, including increased cerebral edema and brain herniation.[11] Thus, these electrolyte imbalances must be effectively corrected and stabilized before transfer to acute care settings.

Hemodynamic Monitoring

Blood pressure goals can vary widely, depending on the neurologic disorder and patient-specific factors and must be stabilized before transfer to acute care units. The ultimate goal is for blood pressure to be maintained at a minimum goal to achieve cerebral perfusion pressure, which corresponds with the patient's best neurologic examination. High blood pressure goals depend on the condition and are reviewed elsewhere in this article.

Blood pressure goals in ischemic stroke are traditionally much higher than in other neurologic conditions to improve collateral circulation. Maximum blood pressure goals depend on the treatment strategy: patients who receive alteplase should have their systolic blood pressure maintained below 180 mm Hg to decrease the risk of hemorrhagic conversion, whereas patients who do not receive alteplase can have a maximum blood pressure goals of 220 mm Hg.[2] Among patients with ischemic stroke, antihypertensive agents are traditionally held, because low blood pressure and accompanying hypoperfusion are also associated with worse outcomes and higher mortality.[13–19] Once neurologic stability is achieved, blood pressure reduction in hypertensive patients can typically be resumed cautiously within 72 hours.[2] When blood pressure reduction is resumed, the health care team should monitor for acute change in neurologic status, but this does not need to occur in the ICU setting.

The optimal blood pressure target in hemorrhagic stroke remains variable. Multiple trials investigating intensive blood pressure lowering and its effect on hematoma expansion and mortality have shown some modest benefit if achieved within 6 hours; however, these studies have failed to show a benefit beyond that time point, with some studies allowing for hypertension up to 180 mm Hg.[20–26]

Hemodynamic targets after aneurysmal subarachnoid hemorrhage are less well-studied, but general recommendations include the maintenance of systolic blood pressure targets at less than 160 mm Hg to prevent the risk of rebleeding.[5,27] Certainly, patient-specific factors and serial neurologic examinations to determine the incidence of vasospasm are important considerations when determining optimal perfusion targets.

Assessing readiness to transfer to the acute care unit from the critical care setting involves an evaluation of the etiology and status of the brain injury, the stabilization of critical parameters, and the ability to successfully deescalate frequent and invasive monitoring modalities. Additional considerations for anticipated length of stay on acute care units, level of care required, and the resources of the receiving unit are also warranted.

Transitioning to Acute Care Units

Once the critical care team has successfully begun the deescalation of ICU care parameters and the patient is deemed appropriate to transfer clinically from the ICU to the acute care unit, clear communication to the receiving clinical team is essential. Up to 80% of errors in hospitals are due to poor communication; risk for these errors increases substantially during handoff between care teams.[28] Errors in handoff can be due to complex underlying physiologic processes, and complex ICU course and complications, placing patients at increased risk for adverse events owing to decreased levels of monitoring, both by personnel and equipment.[29,30]

The integration of specific handoff strategies serves to mitigate the risk of communication errors and ensure the continuity of care during transitions. Specifically, among neuroscience patients transitioning from the ICU to acute care floors, the use of a checklist may significantly decrease communication errors and result in a seamless transition of care and services.[28] Checklist components often include a discussion on medication reconciliation, including current medications, recently discontinued medications, and patient response to opioid and anxiolytic therapies, blood pressure medications, antimicrobials, and anticoagulant therapies, as well as the status of home medications that may have been on hold or need to be resumed before discharge.[28] A discussion should also include line and catheter reconciliation, including the duration and rationale for ongoing need for lines, or the ability to discontinue when appropriate. Strategies for deep vein thrombosis prophylaxis, blood pressure parameters, and pending tests or laboratory values should be included. Last, information on current or anticipated consults should be communicated, including rehabilitation therapies. Patient decision-making capacity, code status, and family contacts and status should be discussed to ensure continuity of communication and discharge planning with key individuals.[28] Physician and nursing handoff should be complementary and interdisciplinary when feasible to ensure the accurate transfer of information between treatment teams.[28]

Wide variation persists among transferring and handoff practices across neurologic settings, which can result in increased ICU readmission rates, medical errors, and adverse events.[31] In addition to standardized checklists, other interventions to optimize the transition of care include the integration of a nurse coordinator to oversee the transfer and communication process from ICU to the floor and to complete the transfer documentation materials.[32,33] Additional strategies include establishing set discharge criteria, use of a bed manager to oversee bed availability and movement, dedicated early discharge planning personnel, the availability of step down unit beds, formalized oversight of medical reconciliation, structured verbal and written handoff techniques and tools, ICU follow-up of discharged patients on the floor, and consulting services or rapid response team that gives floor nurses access to an ICU nurse as a critical resource after ICU discharge.[32] Although no single strategy is associated with decreased ICU readmission, many strategies do improve the transition of care between units and subsequently decrease the risk of medical errors and adverse events.

Predictors for Readmission to the Intensive Care Unit

Although the ultimate goal of transfer to acute care units is to further stabilize the patient in preparation for hospital discharge, patients are at risk for readmission to the ICU after neurologic injury. Readmission to ICU settings after neurologic injury occurs in up to 10% of patients.[33] It is important for interdisciplinary teams to be aware of risk factors for ICU readmission, because there are important considerations for both critical care teams before transfer to acute care floors and for receiving teams managing patients in the acute care setting.

Predictors for ICU readmission among patients with neurologic injury are often not based on transferring practices; rather, the strongest predictors of readmission are based on patient-specific factors.[32] Illness severity scores, such as the Acute Physiology And Chronic Health Evaluation or Simplified Acute Physiology Scores, remain one of the highest predictors if ICU readmission.[34] The presence of high severity scores recorded on ICU admission or discharge are associated with an increased risk of ICU readmission.[35] Each increase in the standard deviation of illness severity scores at these timepoints has been associated with a 43% increased risk of ICU readmission.[35] Additional risk factors across populations include patient comorbidities, age, and the amount of time spent in the ICU.[34–38] Readmission to an ICU is associated with a 10% to 20% increase in patient mortality, double the number of hospital days, and substantial hospital costs.[34] An understanding of the common risk factors can aid in early detection and interventions to decrease ICU readmission from acute care units.

Among patients with neurologic injuries on acute care units, there are often neurologic changes necessitating readmission to ICUs. Common neurologic reasons for ICU readmission include alteration in mental status, need for increased frequency of neurologic assessments, delayed cerebral ischemia, in-hospital stroke, or new-onset or expanding cerebral hemorrhage.[39] Specifically, among neurosurgical patients, complications on acute care units include surgical site infections, bleeding or leakage from surgical sites, seizures, symptomatic cerebral edema or hydrocephalus, infections including sepsis or ventriculitis, and respiratory failure.[39] The most common neurologic indications for ICU readmission include the development of cerebral edema, enlarging cerebral hemorrhage, or seizures.[39]

Although neurologic complications account for 6% to 10% of ICU readmissions, nonneurologic causes account for up to 37% of readmissions.[39] Nonneurologic causes for ICU readmission from acute care units include arrhythmias, cardiac arrest, respiratory failure, renal failure, hyponatremia, hypertension, and hypotension.[39] Respiratory failure and sepsis are the most common causes of ICU readmission.[39] Many of these readmissions occur within 24 to 48 hours of the initial transfer out of the ICU.[39,40]

Specifically, among patients admitted to acute care units after neurologic injury, interdisciplinary teams should consider the initial duration of mechanical ventilation, extubation within 24 hours before transfer, reintubation during ICU stay, and aspiration risk as important factors that could lead to respiratory comprise and subsequent ICU readmission. In addition, the presence of recent seizures, cardiac arrhythmias, hypotensive or hypertensive episodes, increased antibiotic therapies, and recent neurosurgical or radiologic procedure should all warrant close monitoring within acute care units to prevent readmission to the ICU.[40] Interdisciplinary teams should communicate these risks with other care members and family to identify possible strategies to mitigate the risk of complications and ICU readmission. Clear communication of risk can aid in the early detection of deterioration and facilitate timely response to prevent adverse events. The integration of specific risk stratification tools may highlight highest risk areas and prevent ICU readmission.[40]

SUMMARY

The transition of care from the ICU to an acute care unit after critical neurologic injury includes the consideration of a variety of factors to ensure safe and effective care and promote ongoing neurologic recovery. An assessment of the effectiveness of deescalation techniques, agitation management, and risk factor mitigation are important strategies to enhance the success of these transitions. Clear and consistent interdisciplinary communication between teams during handoff between units is imperative to decrease risk of complications, errors, and to streamline discharge processes.

REFERENCES

1. McLaughlin D, Hartjes T, Freeman W. Sleep deprivation in neurointensive care unit patients from serial neurological checks: how much is too much? J Neurosci Nurs 2018;50:205–10.
2. Powers W, Rabinstein AA, Ackerson T, et al. Guidelines for the early management of patients with acute ischemic stroke: a guideline for healthcare professionals from the American Heart Association/American Stroke Association. Stroke 2018;49:e46–99.
3. Sussman ES, Connolly ES. Hemorrhagic transformation: a review of the rate of hemorrhage in the major clinical trials of acute ischemic stroke. Front Neurol 2013;4:69.
4. Hemphill JC, Greenberg SM, Anderson CS, et al. Guidelines for the management of spontaneous intracerebral hemorrhage: a guideline for healthcare professionals from the American Heart Association/American Stroke Association. Stroke 2015;46:2032–60.
5. Connolly ES, Rabinstein AA, Carhuapoma JR, et al. Guidelines for the management of aneursymal subarachnoid hemorrhage: a guideline for healthcare professionals from the American Heart Association/American Stroke Association. Stroke 2012;43:1711–37.
6. Yuan Q, Wu X, Sun Y, et al. Impact of intracranial pressure monitoring on mortality in patients with traumatic brain injury: a systematic review and meta-analysis. J Neurosurg 2015;122:574–87.
7. Ascanio L, Gupta R, Adeeb N, et al. Relationship between external ventricular drain clamp trials and ventriculoperitoneal shunt insertion following nontraumatic subarachnoid hemorrhage: a single-center study. J Neurosurg 2018;16:1–7.
8. Caricato A, Melchionda I, Antonelli M. Continuous electroencephalography monitoring in adults in the intensive care unit. Crit Care 2018;22(1):75.

9. Bleck T. Status epilepticus and the use of continuous EEG monitoring in the intensive care unit. Continuum (Minneap Minn) 2012;18(3):560–78.

10. Ryu J, Walcott BP, Kahle KT, et al. Induced and sustained hypernatremia for the prevention and treatment of cerebral edema following brain injury. Neurocrit Care 2013;19:222–31.

11. Carpenter J, Weinstein S, Myseros J, et al. Inadvertent hyponatremia leading to acute cerebral edema and early evidence of herniation. Neurocrit Care 2007; 6(3):195–9.

12. Qureshi AI, Suarez JI, Bhardwaj A, et al. Use of hypertonic (3%) saline/acetate infusion in the treatment of cerebral edema: effect on intracranial pressure and lateral displacement of the brain. Crit Care Med 1998;26(3):440.

13. Davis MJ, Menon BK, Baghirzada LB, et al. Anesthetic management and outcome in patients during endovascular therapy for acute stroke. Anesthesiology 2012;116:396–405.

14. Mundiyanapurath S, Stehr A, Wolf M, et al. Pulmonary and circulatory parameter guided anesthesia in patients with ischemic stroke undergoing endovascular recanalization. J Neurointerv Surg 2016;8:335–41.

15. Löwhagen Henden P, Rentzos A, Karlsson JE, et al. Hypotension during endovascular treatment of ischemic stroke is a risk factor for poor neurological outcome. Stroke 2015;46:2678–80.

16. Whalin MK, Lopian S, Wyatt K, et al. Dexmedetomidine: a safe alternative to general anesthesia for endovascular stroke treatment. J Neurointerv Surg 2014;6: 270–5.

17. John S, Hazaa W, Uchino K, et al. Lower intraprocedural systolic blood pressure predicts good outcome in patients undergoing endovascular therapy for acute ischemic stroke. Interv Neurol 2016;4:151–7.

18. Whalin MK, Halenda KM, Haussen DC, et al. Even small decreases in blood pressure during conscious sedation affect clinical outcome after stroke thrombectomy: an analysis of hemodynamic thresholds. Am J Neuroradiol 2016. https://doi.org/10.3174/ajnr.A4992.

19. Lee M, Ovbiagele B, Hong KS, et al. Effect of blood pressure lowering in early ischemic stroke: meta-analysis. Stroke 2015;46:1883–9.

20. Butcher KS, Jeerakathil T, Hill M, et al. The intracerebral hemorrhage acutely decreasing arterial pressure trial. Stroke 2013;44:620–6.

21. Anderson CS, Heeley E, Huang Y, et al. Rapid blood-pressure lowering in patients with acute intracerebral hemorrhage. N Engl J Med 2013;368:2355–65.

22. Carcel C, Wang X, Sato S, et al. Degree and timing of intensive blood pressure lowering on hematoma growth in intracerebral hemorrhage: intensive blood pressure reduction in acute cerebral hemorrhage trial-2 results. Stroke 2016;47: 1651–3.

23. Chan E, Anderson CS, Wang X, et al, INTERACT Investigators. Early blood pressure lowering does not reduce growth of intraventricular hemorrhage following acute intracerebral hemorrhage: results of the INTERACT studies. Cerebrovasc Dis Extra 2016;6:71–5.

24. Qureshi AI, Palesch YY, Barsan WG, et al. Intensive blood-pressure lowering in patients with acute cerebral hemorrhage. N Engl J Med 2016;375:1033–43.

25. Steiner T, Al-Shahi Salman R, Beer R, et al. European Stroke Organisation (ESO) guidelines for the management of spontaneous intracerebral hemorrhage. Int J Stroke 2014;9:840–55.

26. McNett M, Moran C, Johnson H. Evidence-based review of clinical trials in neurocritical care. AACN Adv Crit Care 2018;29:195–203.

27. American Association of Neuroscience Nurses. Nursing care of the patient with aneurysmal subarachnoid hemorrhage. Glenview (IL): American Association of Neuroscience Nurses; 2018.

28. Coon EA, Kramer NM, Fabris RR, et al. Structured handoff checklists improve clinical measures in patients discharged from the neurointensive care unit. Neurol Clin Pract 2015;2:42–9.

29. Chaboyer W, Thalib, Foster M, et al. Predictors of adverse events in patients after discharge from the intensive care unit. Am J Crit Care 2008;17:255.

30. Haggstrom M, Asplund K, Kristiansen L. To reduce the technology prior to discharge from intensive care-important but difficult? A grounded theory. Scand J Caring Sci 2013;27:50.

31. Heidegger CP, Treggiari MM, Romand JA. A nationwide survey of intensive care unit discharge practices. Intensive Care Med 2005;31:1676.

32. Van Sluisveld N, Hessselin G, van der Hoeven J, et al. Improving clinical hand-over between intensive care unit and general ward professionals at intensive care unit discharge. Intensive Care Med 2015;41:589–604.

33. Rosenberg AL, Watts C. Patients readmitted to ICUs: a systematic review of risk factors and outcomes. Chest 2000;118:492–502.

34. Wong EG, Parker AM, Leung DG, et al. Association of severity of illness and intensive care unit readmission: a systematic review. Heart Lung 2016;45:3–9.

35. Frost SA, Bogdanovski AE, Salamonson Y, et al. Severity of illness and risk of re-admission to intensive care: a meta-analysis. Resuscitation 2009;80:505–10.

36. Campbell AJ, Cook JA, Adey G, et al. Predicting death and readmission after intensive care discharge. Br J Anesth 2008;100(5):656–62.

37. Duke GJ, Green JV, Briedis JH. Night shift discharge form intensive care unit in-creases the mortality-risk of ICU survivors. Anaesth Intensive Care 2004;32(5): 697–701.

38. Hanane T, Keegan MT, Seferian EG, et al. The association between nighttime transfer from the intensive care unit and patient outcome. Crit Care Med 2008; 36(8):2232–7.

39. Gold CA, Mayer SA, Lennihan L, et al. Unplanned transfers from hospital wards to the neurological intensive care unit. Neurocrit Care 2015;23(2):159–65.

40. Coughlin DG, Kumar MA, Patel NN, et al. Preventing early bouncebacks to the neurointensive care unit: a retrospective analysis and quality improvement pilot. Neurocrit Care 2018;28:175–83.

The Transition from the Hospital to an Inpatient Rehabilitation Setting for Neurologic Patients

Lalita R. Thompson, MSN, RN, CRRN[a], Nneka L. Ifejika, MD, MPH[b],*

KEYWORDS

- Care transition • Rehabilitation • Skilled nursing facility (SNF)
- Inpatient rehabilitation facility (IRF) • Nursing • Physiatry
- Physical medicine and rehabilitation

KEY POINTS

- Transitions of care from acute care hospitals to postacute rehabilitation facilities require a coordinated team approach.
- Early psychiatry/physical medicine and rehabilitation assessment can assist during the acute hospitalization in determining the appropriate level of care.
- Formal partnerships with skilled nursing facilities to improve communication, share clinical knowledge, and engage innovative protocols have the potential to improve patient outcomes.

INTRODUCTION

From the advent of 24-hour acute treatment at comprehensive stroke centers to the continued growth of neurocritical care and interventional neurology, there has been tremendous progress in the care of patients with neurologic diseases. This advancement of health care in the United States has contributed to the improved life expectancy of its citizens. In 1965, the year Medicare was enacted, the life expectancy for white women was 73.7 years; the life expectancy for white men was 66.8 years, and African American life expectancy was approximately 8 to 10 years lower overall than white men. According to the National Vital Statistics 2018 report, the life expectancy of all people in the United States is 78.6 years.[1]

The authors have no industry relationships to disclose.
[a] TiRR Memorial Hermann, 1333 Moursund, Houston, TX 77030, USA; [b] Physical Medicine and Rehabilitation, Neurology and Neurotherapeutics, Population and Data Sciences, University of Texas Southwestern Medical Center, 5323 Harry Hines Boulevard, Dallas, TX 75390-9055, USA
* Corresponding author.
E-mail address: nneka.ifejika@utsouthwestern.edu

Although much attention has been paid to the prolongation of life through acute treatments, less attention has been paid to neurorecovery, particularly, the transition of care from acute hospital settings to postacute rehabilitation. As an example, transitions of care at stroke centers suffer from a lack of standardization, magnified in underinsured populations, and highly variable across health care settings.[2] This lack of standardization is expensive, with a large proportion of this expense attributed to patients with neurologic disease. As an example, between 2012 and 2030, total direct stroke-related costs are expected to triple, from $71.6 billion to $184.1 billion.[3]

In an effort to curb costs, successive changes to the Centers for Medicare and Medicaid Services (CMS) inpatient prospective payment system (PPS) have led to a decrease in the length of acute hospitalization[4–7] and an increase in the use of postacute rehabilitation services,[8] such as inpatient rehabilitation facilities (IRFs) and skilled nursing facilities (SNFs).

Care from an IRF has been correlated with improved outcomes: greater functional recovery,[9–12] higher likelihood of return to the community,[10] and lower rehospitalization rates,[13] compared with care at other settings. Rehabilitation in a SNF has been consistently associated with poor functional outcomes. In an ischemic stroke study, Belagaje and colleagues[14] showed a lower likelihood of good neurologic outcome in stroke patients receiving SNF-based rehabilitation compared with IRF-based rehabilitation after mechanical thrombectomy, despite similar medical severity, neurologic severity, and infarct volume. In a 2006 study of 58,724 Medicare beneficiaries, the odds of community-based discharge were lower for SNF rehabilitation patients with mild to severe motor disabilities after neurologic disease compared with IRF rehabilitation.[9]

The improved quality of care associated with postacute IRF rehabilitation is related to the intensity of professional services. An IRF provides hospital-level care, including 24-hours-a-day rehabilitation nursing, daily physician management, and at least 3 hours of rehabilitation therapy a day, 5 days a week. At SNFs, there is no requirement for direct daily physician contact. A registered nurse (RN) is required for only 8 hours a day, and rehabilitation therapy is provided 1.5 hours a day, 5 days a week.[15] Unfortunately, high-intensity IRF care is associated with higher costs. The median Medicare Part A payment per patient for IRF-based rehabilitation is 40% higher than SNF-based rehabilitation (ie, $23,483 vs $13,472 per stay).[16]

Spasticity, which is experienced in varying degrees, is a common consequence of neurologic disease. The combined effects of pain and impaired function can interfere with patient hygiene, increase fall risk, and decrease quality of life. Although rehabilitation programs at SNFs and IRFs include splints, bracing, and range-of-motion exercises to address spasticity, academic free-standing IRFs traditionally have physiatry-led spasticity management programs, using interventions, such as intramuscular botulinum toxin, phenol injections, and intrathecal baclofen therapy, to further improve functional ability and decrease limb deformity.[17–19]

A 2016 report from the Agency for Healthcare Research and Quality detailed, "no clear guidance exists to determine the type of postacute care setting to which a patient with a specific condition should be discharged."[20] The authors' goal is to detail the transition of care process from the hospital to inpatient rehabilitation settings, obstacles to optimal functional recovery, and future strategies to improve disability rates.

PROSPECTIVE PAYMENT SYSTEM IMPACT ON POSTACUTE QUALITY OF CARE
Skilled Nursing Facility Rehabilitation

In 1983, the CMS instituted the PPS in an effort to lower the costs of health care. The PPS structure reimbursed a predetermined sum based on acute diagnosis and disease severity. As a result, the length of the acute hospital stay decreased, and patients were quickly transitioned to postacute facilities. The initial response of health care systems was the creation of skilled nursing units to care for medically complex patients.[21] The staffing mix included RNs, many with Bachelor of Science in Nursing; physicians rounded on patients with higher frequency, if not daily, and more ancillary services were provided (physical therapy, occupational therapy, speech and language pathology, social work).[21] Medicare reimbursed hospital-based SNFs (HB SNFs) at a higher rate than other SNF types to offset the cost of providing care for higher medical acuity patients. However, the significant cost difference and the rising Medicare expenditure could not be ignored. The Medicare SNF PPS was established in 1998, under which acuity differences between HB SNFs and other SNF types were no longer recognized.[21] Thereafter, all SNFs were reimbursed using the average cost of treating each patient by diagnosis. This new reimbursement structure imposed a significant financial burden on HB SNFs, which was not sustainable. Most SNFs are no longer hospital based.[21]

Hospital-based SNFs were initially established to provide care that is comparable to acute hospitalization, serving as a "way station"[22] between acute care and home. The transfer of neurologically complex patients to nursing home–based SNFs resulted in a considerable loss of nurse management and physician supervision. Strategies to bridge the knowledge gap between HB SNFs and nursing home–based SNFs are essential in the effort to reduce hospital readmissions and improve the quality of patient care.

Inpatient Rehabilitation Facility Rehabilitation

Similar to SNFs, IRFs were historically reimbursed based on the cost of treatment and facility fees.[23] It was not unusual for patients with high cervical complete spinal cord injury to receive treatment at IRFs for up to 6 months, or acute stroke patients to receive treatment for up to 3 months. This extended length of IRF stay afforded the opportunity to receive intensive therapies, family training, and address barriers to returning home.

The CMS 2010 IRF PPS Rule completely modified IRF facility admission criteria. The requirement for patients to potentially tolerate 3 hours of daily physical activity (physical therapy and occupational therapy or speech and language pathology) was instituted,[24] without validation using objective measures of neurologic disease severity. A potential 2-fold negative effect on IRF access ensued. In patients with activity tolerance limitations and for whom skilled nursing services were required to prevent deterioration, rehabilitation at an SNF was recommended. In patients with cognitive greater than physical impairments, home rehabilitation was endorsed. The reduction in length of IRF stay after CMS 2010 resulted in less physical and cognitive gains on the functional independence measure scale, and a decrease in return home rates by 5.4%.[23,25]

TRANSITIONS OF CARE BARRIERS

The implementation of CMS cost savings in the postacute realm created a domino effect regarding access to rehabilitation care. Patients in Medicare Health Maintenance Organizations or managed care plans are more likely to receive postacute rehabilitation services at SNF rather than IRF rehabilitation when compared with patients with traditional Medicare fee-for-service plans.[26] Many state Medicaid plans do not cover IRF or SNF rehabilitation, leaving low-income patients with neurologic disease without a postacute rehabilitation option. There is a growing trend for providers and hospitals to not accept Medicaid-managed care plans, and traditional Medicaid in some states only extends to children under the age of 21, further increasing health disparities for low-income populations.[27,28]

Geography is another barrier to patients with neurologic disease receiving postacute rehabilitation care. There are approximately 1,188 IRFs and 15,080 SNFs in the United States,[29] and IRFs are mainly in states with high populations of Medicare recipients. It is reasonable to deduce that some patients who are appropriate for IRF rehabilitation may be transitioned to a nearby SNF for rehabilitation care; indeed, the proximity of the SNF to home can prove convenient for the patient and their family. A qualitative study done by Tyler and colleagues[30] showed most acute care hospitals provide a list of SNFs to patients/families within the geographic area but shy away from providing additional information regarding intensity of therapies, acute readmission rates, or community discharge rates, for fear of violating the Stark Law. The proximity of the SNF to home leads the reason patient and family choose SNF. Without sufficient information on SNF quality measures, patients/families often choose low-quality SNF based on location.[31] The Stark Law was enacted to prevent the unethical practice of physician self-referrals of Medicare and Medicaid recipients to facilities, services, or other health care professionals for which the physician has a financial relationship.[32] Physician self-referrals limited patient choice to entities that provided a monetary "kickback" to the physician. Violations of the Stark Law extend back to the affiliated hospital organization, and penalties can cost organizations substantial sums, including denial of the acute care hospitalization.[33] Essentially, the Stark Law hinders the ability of health care providers to guide patients toward higher-quality facilities.[34,35]

OPPORTUNITIES TO IMPROVE TRANSITIONS OF CARE FROM THE ACUTE HOSPITAL TO POSTACUTE REHABILITATION

The code of ethics for physicians, nurses, and other health care professionals includes the phrase "do no harm." The transition of patients with neurologic disease from acute to postacute care facilities requires a coordinated approach focused on safety. This coordinated approach includes physicians, nursing, case management, social work, physical therapy, occupational therapy, and speech and language pathology in both realms. Poor communication between acute care and postacute care team creates the opportunity for errors.[36,37] The Joint Commission Sentinel Event Alert 58 exposed preventable avoidable errors if adequate communication of crucial information was exchanged.[38] The use of standardized communication tools can guide telephone handoff between acute care physician and nurse and receiving postacute facility physician and nurse.[38–41] An electronic handoff form should include critical information, such as medications, allergies, treatments, diagnosis, significant past medical history, pending tests, and functional status. A standardized form should provide structured communication to decrease errors but not hinder open dialogue and exchange of information. Communication of contact information for the nursing unit and attending physician ranked high priority among SNF nurses that participated in a qualitative study.[37]

The responsibility of evaluating the postacute care facility capacity to manage the patient is incumbent on the acute care hospital or sending facility.[42] Preparation for care transition includes the knowledge of patient-centered outcomes. The creation of informative postacute referral lists can provide guidance, without impeding on patient choice and unintentionally violating the Stark Law. For each postacute rehabilitation facility near the acute hospital and the patient's home, documentation of nursing staff mix (RN, licensed vocational nurse), nurse-to-patient ratio, quality star rating, services offered, and physician coverage[21,30] are recommended.

Find a Physiatrist

The critical barrier between transitioning patients with neurologic disease from acute care to IRF rehabilitation is a lack of recognition of the patient's rehabilitation potential. Physiatrists have an established leadership role in IRFs, by means of their extensive training in rehabilitation, impairment, and function.[43] Physiatry consultation at the acute care hospital to assist in the evaluation of rehabilitation needs, including synthesis of physician, nursing, physical therapy, occupational therapy, and speech and language pathology assessments, and appropriateness for IRF or SNF care can improve the transition. Furthermore, limited knowledge of postacute care regulations by the primary acute care team may delay or preclude transition to the appropriate level of care when communicating with an authorization representative at the insurance company.[42] Physiatry, as a medical specialty, focuses on the "diagnoses, evaluation, and management of persons of all ages with physical and/or cognitive impairments, disabilities, and functional limitations."[44]

Gear Up for Skilled Nursing Facilities

It is imperative that health care professionals educate patients and their families about SNFs to guide their decision-making process. In addition, clinicians must form better relationships with SNFs to formulate and implement strategies to improve SNF care. For patients transitioning from an acute care hospital to an SNF for rehabilitation, there are opportunities to bridge the gap and potentially improve patient outcomes.

- *Supplemental activities:* IRF rehabilitation centers provide primarily out-of-bed therapy services 3 hours daily, 5 days a week. Indeed, physiatrists often journey to the therapy gym to complete daily physician assessments. The SNFs may not have access to therapy gyms with advanced technology; however, family training in transfers, range-of-motion, and bed level exercises by physical therapy and occupational therapies at SNFs can not only improve activity tolerance but also decrease the risks of contracture and development of spasticity. In addition, review of the orthotic-wearing schedule, stretching techniques, proper splint placement, and education on signs of skin breakdown can also help prepare for eventual transition to home.

- *Early communication:* In the age of electronic medical record systems, there are pages of information that is repetitive and not immediately useful. Verbal communication is a key in the transition process. Once the next level of care has been determined, the acute care hospital nurse should contact the IRF or SNF rehabilitation nursing staff 24 hours in advance to help ease the transition of care process. Confirmation of access to prescribed medications, feeding tube formulation and supplies (if applicable), tracheostomy management, wound care, and nursing interventions in advance can prepare the staff for the patient's specific needs. This is especially important for nonverbal patients. Transferring a patient to postacute care with unused enteral formula and supplies from the day of discharge can allow time for the postacute facility to obtain items, resulting in heightened care continuity. In addition, the receiving facility should have information on whom to contact in the event there are any questions. Communication of the patient's acuity level and the use of patient assignment algorithms can help improve nursing care inequities at centers with high patient volume. Rehab MATRIX, piloted by certified rehabilitation registered nurses (CRRNs) at a hospital-based IRF in Houston, Texas, is a nursing-led tool that equitable assigns newly admitted IRF patients using select acuity variables. [45]

TRANSITION TO OUTPATIENT NEUROREHABILITATION SERVICES

Patients are most vulnerable to readmission during care transitions from postacute rehabilitation to the community. Outpatient rehabilitation is an important component on the neurorehabilitation continuum, serving as a bridge between the inpatient rehabilitation stay and home.[42] A comprehensive outpatient rehabilitation program for patients with neurologic disease should include physical therapy, occupational therapy, and speech and language pathology to advance the functional improvements made during the inpatient rehabilitation hospitalization, outpatient rehabilitation clinic care with physiatry social work services, and CRRN feedback to improve education on outpatient medications.

Medication compliance is an important part of the community transition for patients with neurologic disease. Rehabilitation nursing can not only provide medication education to caregivers and family while hospitalized but also ensure those medications have been dispensed to the patient after discharge. Some rehabilitation facilities call patients 24 to 48 hours after discharge, weekly for 30 days, until the outpatient follow-up clinic appointment. This consistent contact helps relieve patient/family anxiety and provides early identification of concerns that may lead to readmissions or emergency room visits.[46] A common complaint of patients and caregivers is the requirement for preauthorization for outpatient medications. Several days can pass before insurance approval, leading to a gap in treatment. Nursing collaboration with pharmacy services and initiation of the prior authorization process several days in advance of community discharge may lead to fewer delays. The cost of medication or the copayment amount can also increase the likelihood of noncompliance. Case management identification of high-cost medications, combined with pharmacy determination of viable alternatives and social work identification of available resources to assist with copayments, can provide multiple levels of assistance.

Adaptive equipment is an important part of returning home after rehabilitation care. Unfortunately, ill-fitting equipment, such as rented wheelchairs and lifts, which do not provide total body weight support, are common obstacles that patients with neurologic disease have to overcome. Furthermore, delivery delays to home for proper fitting equipment often result from ineffective care coordination.[42,47] Inpatient practice sessions using appropriate lift transfer equipment can decrease patient stress and mitigate caregiver anxiety. Nursing collaboration with the therapy team for patient follow-up calls to address equipment issues can also prove beneficial.

Medicare beneficiaries with neurologic disease faced another financial barrier to reaching maximal functional improvement: therapy limitations. In 2017, the therapy cap was maximized at $2,010 annually, with physical therapy and speech therapy sharing the therapy cap per calendar year.[48] Occupational therapy has the full amount per calendar year. When Medicare decreases therapy reimbursements, the potential response of health care organizations is to limit services, decrease the cost of supplies, and increase employee responsibilities. These adjustments may delay initiation of outpatient therapy services and decrease the frequency of therapy visits.

Effective and conscientious case management and social work services can identify obstacles such as lack of transportation[42,49] and determine lower-cost therapy providers in the community. In the current inpatient rehabilitation care model, IRF and SNF case management concentrates on maximizing resources during the insurance company–authorized hospitalization. The focus of social work services is primarily on discharge disposition (ie, Does the patient have somewhere to go? Is there an identified caregiver?). Reframing the role of case management and social work to think past the acute rehabilitation stay, and on to the weeks and months thereafter, is an opportunity for future development.

SUMMARY

Transitions of care from acute care hospitals to postacute rehabilitation facilities require a coordinated team approach. With the trend to further reduce acute hospital length of stay and decrease health care costs, innovative paradigms are needed to heighten functional improvements, decrease readmissions, and improve community discharge rates. Early physiatry assessment can assist during the acute hospitalization in determining the appropriate level of care. Formal partnerships with SNFs to improve communication, share clinical knowledge, and engage innovative protocols have the potential to improve patient outcomes.

Nurses play an integral role on the acute care and rehabilitation care teams; however, there is a need for substantial expansion. Nurses spend the most time with patients preparing them for discharge readiness through education and patient-centered care interventions. Nurses are involved in follow-up calls to the patient after discharge to home; however, how many acute care hospitals call postacute facilities after discharge to make sure all is well? Discharge follow-up calls to post-acute facility 24 to 48 hours after discharge from acute care hospital provides the ability to identify and address unanticipated barriers. Nurses can no longer view hospital discharge as the end of patient care; they must remain actively involved during the transition period. In the rehabilitation setting, the use of RNs within a comprehensive rehabilitation clinic for telephone triage can assist the patient's transition to home. Rehabilitation nursing is centered on providing safe, efficient, holistic, patient-centered care to improve the lives of those with disabilities. CRRNs have the training, education, and governing authority to assess and triage patients to identify actual and potential problems. This role has the potential to evolve into an inpatient rehabilitation nurse navigator, bridging the gap between the inpatient and outpatient realm.

ACKNOWLEDGMENTS

Current Funding: Dr N.L. Ifejika - Texas Health Resources Clinical Scholars Program – UT Southwestern. Prior Funding: Dr N.L. Ifejika - NIH/NCATS McGovern Medical School at UTHealth CCTS Scholar UL1 TR000371; NIH/NINDS Diversity Supplement to P50 NS 044227, UTHSC-Houston Specialized Program of Translational Research in Acute Stroke (SPOTRIAS).

REFERENCES

1. Xu JQ, Murphy SL, Kochanek KD, et al. Deaths: final data for 2016. National Vital Statistics reports, vol. 67. Hyattsville (MD): National Center for Health Statistics; 2018. 5.
2. Broderick JP, Abir M. Transitions of care for stroke patients: opportunities to improve outcomes. Circ Cardiovasc Qual Outcomes 2015;8(6 Suppl 3): S190–2.
3. Ovbiagele B, Goldstein LB, Higashida RT, et al. Forecasting the future of stroke in the United States: a policy statement from the American Heart Association and American Stroke Association. Stroke 2013;44:2361–75.

4. Hall MJ, Levant S, DeFrances CJ. Hospitalization for stroke in U.S. hospitals, 1989–2009. NCHS data brief, no 95. Hyattsville (MD): National Center for Health Statistics; 2012. Available at: https://www.cdc.gov/nchs/data/databriefs/db95.pdf.

5. Benjamin EJ, Virani SS, Callaway CW, et al. Heart disease and stroke statistics—2018 update: a report from the American Heart Association. Circulation 2018; 137:e67.

6. Levant S, Chari K, DeFrances CJ. Hospitalizations for patients aged 85 and over in the United States, 2000–2010. NCHS data brief, no 182. Hyattsville (MD): National Center for Health Statistics; 2015. Available at: https://www.cdc.gov/nchs/data/databriefs/db182.pdf.

7. Ramirez L, Kim-Tenser MA, Sanossian N, et al. Trends in acute ischemic stroke hospitalizations in the United States. J Am Heart Assoc 2016;5 [pii:e003233].

8. Gage B. Impact of the BBA on post-acute utilization. Health Care Financ Rev 1999;20:103–26.

9. Deutsch A, Granger CV, Heinemann AW, et al. Poststroke rehabilitation: outcomes and reimbursement of inpatient rehabilitation facilities and subacute rehabilitation programs. Stroke 2006;37:1477–82.

10. Kramer AM, Steiner JF, Schlenker RE, et al. Outcomes and costs after hip fracture and stroke: a comparison of rehabilitation settings. JAMA 1997;277:396–404.

11. Kane RL, Chen Q, Finch M, et al. Functional outcomes of posthospital care for stroke and hip fracture patients under Medicare. J Am Geriatr Soc 1998;46: 1525–33.

12. Keith RA, Wilson DB, Gutierrez P. Acute and subacute rehabilitation for stroke: a comparison. Arch Phys Med Rehabil 1995;76:495–500.

13. Prvu Bettger J, Liang L, Xian Y, et al. Inpatient rehabilitation facility care reduces the likelihood of death and re-hospitalization after stroke compared with skilled nursing facility care. Stroke 2015;46:A146 [abstract].

14. Belagaje SR, Sun CJ, Nogueira RG, et al. Discharge disposition to skilled nursing facility after endovascular reperfusion therapy predicts a poor prognosis. J Neurointerv Surg 2015;7(2):99–103.

15. Buntin MB. Access to postacute rehabilitation. Arch Phys Med Rehabil 2007;88: 1488–93.

16. Buntin MB, Colla CH, Deb P, et al. Medicare spending and outcomes after post-acute care for stroke and hip fracture. Med Care 2010;48(9):776–84.

17. Bakheit AMO. The pharmacological management of post-stroke muscle spasticity. Drugs Aging 2012;29:941–7.

18. Kuo C, Hu G. Post-stroke spasticity: a review of epidemiology, pathophysiology, and treatments. Int J Gerontol 2018;12:280–4.

19. Saulino M, Guillemette S, Leier J, et al. Medical cost impact of intrathecal baclofen therapy for severe spasticity. Neuromodulation 2015;18:141–9.

20. Tian W. An all-payer view of hospital discharge to postacute care, 2013. Healthcare Cost and Utilization Project Statistical Brief #205. Rockville (MD): Agency for Healthcare Research and Quality; 2016. Available at: https://www.hcup-us.ahrq.gov/reports/statbriefs/sb205-Hospital-Discharge-Postacute-Care.pdf. Accessed January 15, 2019.

21. Rahman M, Zinn JS, Mor V. The impact of hospital-based skilled nursing facility closures on rehospitalizations. Health Serv Res 2013;48:499–518.

22. Morris JN, Berg K, Topinkova E, et al. Developing quality indicators for in-patient post-acute care. BMC Geriatr 2018;18. https://doi.org/10.1186/s12877-018-0842-z.

23. Dobrez D, Heinemann AW, Deutsch A, et al. Impact of Medicare's prospective payment system for inpatient rehabilitation facilities on stroke patient outcomes. Am J Phys Med Rehabil 2010;89:198–204.
24. Gage B, Smith L, Coots L, et al. Analysis of the classification criteria for inpatient rehabilitation facilities (IRFs) 2009. CMS Contract No. HHSM-500-2009-0002G. Available at: https://www.cms.gov/InpatientRehabFacPPS/Downloads/RTC_Analysis_Classification_Criteria_IRF.pdf. Accessed January 15, 2019.
25. O'Brien SR, Xue Y, Ingersoll G, et al. Shorter length of stay is associated with worse functional outcomes for Medicare beneficiaries with stroke. Phys Ther 2013;93:1592–602.
26. Higashida R, Alberts MJ, Alexander DN, et al. Interactions within stroke systems of care: a policy statement from the American Heart Association/American Stroke Association. Stroke 2013;44:2961–84.
27. Renter E. You've got Medicaid—why can't you see the doctor? U.S News and World Report 2015 (Online). Available at: https://health.usnews.com/health-news/health-insurance/articles/2015/05/26/youve-got-medicaid-why-cant-you-see-the-doctor.
28. Bindman AB, Coffman JM. Calling all doctors: what type of insurance do you accept? JAMA Intern Med 2014;174(6):869–70.
29. Medicare Payment Advisory Commission (MedPAC) report to the congress: Medicare payment policy. 2018. Available at: http://www.medpac.gov/docs/default-source/reports/mar18_medpac_entirereport_sec.pdf.
30. Tyler DA, Gadbois EA, McHugh JP, et al. Patients are not given quality-of-care data about skilled nursing facilities when discharged from hospitals. Health Aff (Millwood) 2017;36:1385–91.
31. Rahman M, McHugh J, Gozalo PL, et al. The contribution of skilled nursing facilities to hospitals' readmission rate. Health Serv Res 2017;52:656–75.
32. Tharp J. Stark Law and the affordable care act: bridging the disconnect. J Leg Med 2014;35:433–44.
33. Collins A, Clark K, George AA. Stark future for the Stark Law? Home Healthc Now 2018;36(6):393.
34. Rahman M, Grabowski DC, Mor V, et al. Is a skilled nursing facility's rehospitalization rate a valid quality measure? Health Serv Res 2016;51(6):2158–75.
35. Finnegan J. Groups back Stark Law changes to eliminate barrier to value-based models. Fierce Healthcare 2018.
36. Dambaugh L, Ecklund MM. Transitional care: assuring evidence-based practice in skilled nursing facilities. Clin Nurse Spec 2014;28:315–7.
37. King BJ, Gilmore-Bykovskyi AL, Roiland RA, et al. The consequences of poor communication during transitions from hospital to skilled nursing facility: a qualitative study. J Am Geriatr Soc 2013;61:1095–102.
38. Tomsky N. Communication breakdown: sentinel event alert calls out bad patient handoffs. Briefings on Accreditation and Quality. American Nurses Credentialing Center (ANCC) 2018;29(1):7–11.
39. The Joint Commission Center for Transforming Healthcare. Targeted solutions Tool® for hand-off communications. Oakbrook Terrace (IL): The Joint Commission; 2017.
40. Rosenthal JL, Doiron R, Haynes SC, et al. The effectiveness of standardized handoff tool interventions during inter- and intra-facility care transitions on patient-related outcomes: a systematic review. Am J Med Qual 2018;33:193–206.
41. Hill CE, Varma P, Lenrow D, et al. Reducing errors in transition from acute stroke hospitalization to inpatient rehabilitation. Front Neurol 2015;6:227.

42. Camicia M, Black T, Farrell J, et al. The essential role of the rehabilitation nurse in facilitating care transitions: a white paper by the association of rehabilitation nurses. Rehabil Nurs 2014;39(1):3–15.

43. Laker SR, Adair WA 3rd, Annaswamy TM, et al. American Academy of Physical Medicine and Rehabilitation position statement on definitions for rehabilitation physician and director of rehabilitation in inpatient rehabilitation settings. PM R 2019;11:98–102.

44. Accreditation Council for Graduate Medical Education (ACGME). ACGME program requirements for graduate medical education in physical medicine and rehabilitation. Available at: https://www.acgme.org/Portals/0/PFAssets/Program Requirements/340_physical_medicine_rehabilitation_2017-07-01.pdf. Accessed December 7, 2018.

45. Ifejika NL, Okpala MN, Moser HA, et al. Rehab MATRIX: content validity of a nursing-led patient assignment algorithm. J Neurosci Nurs 2019;51:33–6.

46. Harrison JD, Auerbach AD, Quinn K, et al. Assessing the impact of nurse post-discharge telephone calls on 30-day hospital readmission rates. J Gen Intern Med 2014;29:1519–25.

47. Lutz BJ, Young ME, Creasy KR, et al. Improving stroke caregiver readiness for transition from inpatient rehabilitation to home. Gerontologist 2017;57:880.

48. American Occupational Therapy Association. Full repeal of outpatient Medicare therapy cap signed into law. Physical Therapy Products (Online) 2018.

49. Fahlberg B. Preventing readmissions through transitional care. Nursing 2017; 47:12–4.

Understanding the Experience of Early Supported Discharge from the Perspective of Patients with Stroke and Their Carers and Health Care Providers
A Qualitative Review

Candice L. Osborne, PhD, MPH, OTR[a],*, Marsha Neville, PhD, OTR[b]

KEYWORDS

- Continuity of patient care • Transitional care • Research • Stroke • Rehabilitation
- Neurologic rehabilitation • Patient care

KEY POINTS

- A qualitative review of the early supported discharge (ESD) experience revealed 2 main themes: psychosocial aspects of ESD and the experience of the logistical components of the process.
- Patient, carer, and providers valued the relationships that formed during the ESD intervention.
- Communication played a significant role in the overall experience of ESD.
- The home environment provides a familiar space where patients can return to roles and routines and providers can tailor treatment sessions to meet the needs of the patients.

INTRODUCTION

After a stroke, patients and those close to them inevitably experience major shifts in roles, responsibilities, and life plans. The course of treatment can include acute hospitalization and rehabilitation. Rehabilitation traditionally includes inpatient therapy

The authors of this article have no commercial or financial conflicts of interest.
[a] Department of Physical Medicine and Rehabilitation, University of Texas Southwestern Medical Center, CS6.110 Charles Sprague Building, 5161 Harry Hines Boulevard, Dallas, TX 75390, USA; [b] Department of Occupational Therapy, School of Occupational Therapy, Texas Woman's University, 5500 Southwestern Medical Avenue, Dallas, TX 75235, USA
* Corresponding author.
E-mail address: Candice.osborne@utsouthwestern.edu

often followed by outpatient therapy or therapy delivered in the home. Early supported discharge (ESD) is a model of health care delivery reducing lengths of hospital stay with accelerated discharge home after a stroke. ESD enables persons with mild to moderate impairments and a capable support system to return home sooner and receive therapies within the familiar surroundings of home. Evidence suggests that early therapy in the home is beneficial,[1] because patients and carers experience real-world practice as opposed to rehabilitation intervention in the hospital, where tasks can only be simulated. ESD allows for problem solving and planning in context. Performing real tasks in the home rather than simulating the tasks in an unfamiliar environment is motivating and makes the intervention relevant to individuals and the carers.

To examine the experience of ESD from the perspective of persons with stroke, carers, and health care personnel, a systematic review of qualitative evidence was conducted. Qualitative research methods have been described as an interpretive, naturalistic approach for exploring the perspectives of research participants for the purpose of understanding a phenomena. The aims and objectives of qualitative research are to provide an in-depth understanding of the experiences of the participants.[2] Data derived from interviews, observation, and/or immersion in an experience are the basis for secondary analysis of the depth and complexity of the studied phenomena.

METHODS
Search Strategy

The authors performed a comprehensive search of 3 databases (MEDLINE, CINAHL, and Embase) with a search strategy developed in MEDLINE and adapted for the remaining databases. The search strategy included relevant subject headings (Medical Subject Headings [MeSH]) and Boolean logic search terms, OR and AND, with no date restrictions. Publications were limited to English language. Reference lists also were scanned to identify relevant publications (**Box 1**. The primary aim of this review is to explore the experience of ESD from the perspectives of patients, carers, and their health care providers.

Study Types

Studies included were published in peer-reviewed journals and used qualitative methods of data collection, such as focus groups, interviews, and/or surveys that contained open-ended/descriptive response items. Mixed-method studies were included if the qualitative data could be extracted. Studies were excluded if (1) they included patient populations other than stroke, (2) there was no examination of patient/carer/health care professional (hospital or community based) perspectives of ESD, or (3) they examined a program other than ESD.

Study Participants

Studies were eligible for inclusion if the study participants were (1) adults (over 18 years old) with a diagnosis of stroke who were discharged from hospital-based acute care to home as part of an ESD program, (2) adult care partners (unpaid carers, such as spouses or partners, family members, friends, or significant others, who provide physical or emotional support) of patients with stroke discharged home as part of an ESD program, and (3) health care professionals (both hospital based and community based) who provided services to patients with stroke as part of the an ESD program. ESD was defined as rehabilitation

Box 1
Search strategy for MEDLINE

Database: Ovid MEDLINE(R) <1946 to October 25, 2018>, Ovid MEDLINE(R) In-Process & Other Non-Indexed Citations <October 25, 2018>, Ovid MEDLINE(R) Epub Ahead of Print <October 25, 2018>

1. "early supported discharge".tw. (130)
2. Stroke Rehabilitation/ (11223)
3. exp Stroke/th [Therapy] (11797)
4. Patient Discharge/ (25931)
5. Home care services/ (31603)
6. ("home based rehabilitation" or "home rehabilitation").tw. (576)
7. 1 or 4 (26001)
8. 2 or 3 (22165)
9. 5 or 6 (32008)
10. 7 and 8 and 9 (73)
11. Limit 10 to English language (69)
12. exp Qualitative Research/ (42128)
13. qualitative.tw. (190889)
14. 12 or 13 (203881)
15. 11 and 14 (8)
16. Limit 11 to "qualitative (best balance of sensitivity and specificity)" (16)
17. exp Cohort Studies/ (1790959)
18. Observational Study/ (53767)
19. Focus Groups/ (25484)
20. exp INTERVIEW, PSYCHOLOGICAL/ or exp INTERVIEW/ (42815)
21. 17 or 18 or 19 or 20 (1872512)
22. 11 and 21 (26)
23. Limit 11 to observational study (2)
24. 15 or 16 or 22 or 23 (40)
25. ("observational" or "focus group*" or interview*).tw. (472362)
26. stroke.tw. (209007)
27. 1 and 26 (102)
28. 13 or 25 (595392)
29. 27 and 28 (19)
30. 29 not 24 (10)
31. From 30 keep 1–6, 10 (7)
32. 24 or 31 (47)

that (1) takes place in a patient's home environment and (2) replaces inpatient rehabilitation after the acute phase of stroke. Early stroke management can vary by country or region. Therefore, for the purpose of this analysis, the acute care setting includes hospital-based initial inpatient care, specialized stroke treatment facilities, and step-down hospital settings.

Data Collection

Using the preestablished screening criteria, 1 reviewer (CLO) screened titles, abstracts, and full-text articles resulting from the database searches. Data were extracted from each eligible article by CLO and were compared against the original article by MN. Extracted data included (1) country, (2) study type (focus group, interview, questionnaire, etc.), (3) participants (ie, patients, care partners, and health care professionals), (4) qualitative themes identified in each study, and (5) program description. In addition, each eligible study was scored separately by the reviewers (MN and CLO) using the Critical Appraisal Skills Programme (CASP),[3] a quality assessment based on Cochrane guidelines[4] that guides the appraisal of the rationale for the study method, data analysis, and key findings as well as ethical considerations and overall value of the research. CASP scoring disagreements were resolved through discussion.

Synthesis

Narrative synthesis was used to identify key concepts across studies. All included studies were read and reread, and key concepts were listed for each. Concepts were coded and the coded data then were merged and categorized by topic and subtopic using matrices to organize and compare the data to identity emerging patterns. Summaries of findings were created and review by the authors.[5]

RESULTS
Study Selection

The search resulted in 160 citations; 13 were duplicate citations. Therefore, 147 citations were identified. Citations were reviewed according to the Preferred Reporting Items for Systematic Reviews and Meta-Analyses (PRISMA) standards (see **Fig. 1** for PRISMA flow diagram). Sixteen full-text citations were screened and 6 studies met inclusion criteria[6–12] (the results of 1 study are described in 2 separate articles;

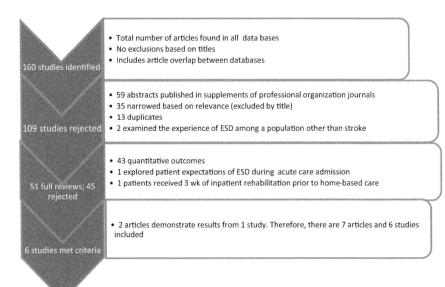

Fig. 1. PRISMA flow diagram.

both articles are included in this review[6,7]). In 1 case, providers, patients, and carers who experienced the ESD process were interviewed separately, resulting in 2 separate studies of the same intervention (providers in 1 and patients and carers in the other). They are included as 2 separate studies in this review.[11,12]

Studies were excluded most commonly due to (1) study type—a majority of studies identified were quantitative and did not include qualitative outcomes; (2) abstract only with no article—a majority of citations identified in the Embase database were abstracts published in supplements of professional organization journals; (3) setting—several qualitative studies examined the hospital discharge experience of conventional discharge routines, not of ESD programs; and (4) population—2 of the studies examined the experience of ESD among a population other than stroke (i.e. chronic obstructive pulmonary disease).

Study Details

All the studies used a face-to-face interview design. Three of the studies had between 28 and 40 participants[10–12] and 3 studies were smaller, with 4 to 8 participants in each.[6–9] Two studies were interviews conducted among ESD care providers,[9,11] 2 were interviews conducted among patients who experienced ESD,[6–8] and 2 were interviews conducted among patients who experienced ESD and their carers.[10,12] Interviews among patients and carers in all studies were conducted no later than 8 months post-stroke but took place at varying times during those 8 months. In all but 1 of the studies that included patients and/or carers, interviews were conducted after the ESD intervention had concluded.[6–8,10] Three of the 6 studies included a description of the ESD intervention.[9–11] Qualitative analysis varied across each of the studies included, but all studies conducted a standardized qualitative analysis and thematic synthesis (**Table 1**).

Quality Appraisal

Based on the results of the Critical Appraisal Skills Programme (CASP): quality assessment tool, the methodology and overall quality of each of the studies were moderate to good (**Table 2**). All the studies reported a clear purpose, and the use of qualitative versus quantitative methodology was appropriate based on the stated objective of each of the studies. Two of the studies did not justify their use of the chosen study design,[9,11] and 1 study did not meet criteria for appropriate recruitment strategy because the investigators did not disclose why a willing study participant who met inclusion criteria was not selected for an interview.[8]

One of the most frequent overall study quality deficits was in the area of data collection; 3 studies did not address saturation of data.[6–8,11] Therefore, it is unclear whether or not the data collected are robust and/or applicable to others who have experienced ESD or provided care within an ESD model. A second study quality deficit was lack of exploration of the relationship between the interviewer and the participants. Only 1 of the 6 studies acknowledged and discussed the impact of this relationship.[6,7] The background of the interviewer and whether or not the interviewer has an established relationship with the interviewee can influence how questions are asked, what content is pursued during the discussion, and how forthcoming an interviewee may be with personal thoughts or opinions. These potential biases may influence the data collected in the studies included in this review.

Thematic Findings

The synthesis of qualitative data collected for the purpose of understanding the experience of ESD revealed 2 main themes. The first was the psychosocial aspects of ESD. This theme included 2 subthemes: (1) the emotional experience of ESD and (2) the

Table 1
Study characteristics

Author/Country	Study Type	Participants	Data Analysis	Key Findings/General Conclusions	Purpose of the Study	Program Description
Taule and Raheim,[6] 2014 Norway	Face-to-face interview in an RCT	Patients 6–8 mo post–mild stroke (n = 8) recruited from a larger RCT of conventional treatment vs ESD	Interpretive description supplemented with systematic text condensation	The Taule and colleagues articles included in this review (2014 and 2015) report results from the same study in 2 articles. Core theme: "life changed existentially." Subthemes were (1) self-perceived health; (2) a changed body; (3) performing ADLs and work; (4) taking part in society: freedom and loss; and (5) self-perception.	Patient-attributed meanings of activity and participation in the home recovery process (existential dimensions of the participants' stories)	None given; part of RCT? = yes
Chouliara et al,[11] 2014 England	Face-to-face interview	Staff working in ESD-relevant job role at 2 separate hospitals in Nottinghamshire England (n = 35)	Data were coded and categorized, then collapsed into frequent key themes by 2 separate researchers. Differences were discussed and resolved.	Facilitators for ESD—adaptability of the intervention to the health care context, support from rehabilitation assistance, collaboration among services; ESD challenges—unclear referral process, fragmented stroke pathway, assessment	Explores perceptions of health care professionals regarding (1) the challenges and facilitators to implementing an evidence-based service and (2) the perceived impact of ESD services	Multidiscipline, 1–2 interventions/d, 7 d/wk, for up to 6 wk; part of RCT? = no

Collins et al,[8] 2016 Ireland	Face-to-face interview	Patients who experienced ESD (n = 4) Patients were 2 wk to 3 mo post-discharge from ESD	Frequently recurrent concepts were classified as themes. Two authors completed coding and discrepancies were resolved through discussion.	duplication; impact of ESD—patient-centered intervention, reduced hospital stay, smoother transition from hospital to home Hospital discharge is a significant milestone and an anxiety-inducing time; rehabilitation in a familiar environment (home) is more meaningful; patients did not demonstrate clear insight regarding ESD; positive social aspect—relationship between provider and patient in the home environment	Explores the experiences of ESD from the perspective of stroke survivors	None given; part of RCT? = no
Cobley et al,[12] 2013 England	Face-to-face interview	Patients (n = 27, 19 experienced ESD) and carer (n = 15, 9 experienced ESD) who experienced or were eligible for ESD (2-group comparison); 1 mo to 6 mo post-discharge	Thematic analysis; relevance of each them was assessed by a second researcher; differences were discussed and agreement was reached.	Patients and carer: home environment allows for a tailored intervention, more privacy; majority of carer satisfied with respite during sessions; majority reported a seamless transition from hospital to home, but felt care ended abruptly at 6 wk and	Explores patients and carers perceptions of ESD services during the early post-discharge phase	None given; part of RCT? = no

(continued on next page)

Table 1
(continued)

Author/Country	Study Type	Participants	Data Analysis	Key Findings/General Conclusions	Purpose of the Study	Program Description
				they were ill prepared; carer only: felt ill prepared for new role and unsupported—lack of education, training, and information		
Taule et al,[7] 2015 Norway	Face-to face interview in an RCT	Patients with mild stroke who experienced ESD (n = 8); data collected 6–8 mo poststroke	Interpretive description supplemented with systematic text condensation	Processing emotions about the impact physical and cognitive changes—feelings of isolation; the impact of the provider-patient relationship dynamics—a balance between optimism and realism; impact of unclear information/training; negative impact of abrupt end to ESD with lag time between EDS care and community-based care	Explores mild to moderate stroke survivors' experience with home rehabilitation after ESD	None given; part of RCT? = yes
Lou et al,[10] 2016 Denmark	Face-to-face interview	Patients who experienced ESD (n = 22) and their care partners (n = 18): data collected 3 wk–6 wk after stroke	Thematic analysis; themes organized in a thematic map were investigated in relation to the full	Patients and carers felt ill-informed; home as place of calmness and privacy compared with hospital; home was a place of meaningful	Investigate how mild stroke patients and their partners experience and manage life in the context of ESD.	Stroke team assesses 2–7 d post-discharge. Treats patients for 1–4 visits; part of RCT? = no

| von Koch et al,[9] 2000 Sweden | Face-to-face interview design | Participants (OT, PT, speech) who worked in an ESD | Step-by-step procedure of separate analysis of each interview, themes and categories discussed for consensus. data set and final themes were defined. | Importance of being a good listener; patient-centered goals; problem-solving strategies; therapist-patient relationship; visit frequency; understanding desires, abilities, environmental demands and expectations; carer model; therapy in hospital vs home; partnership activity; maintaining hope for recovery; provider-patient-carer relationship may be more equitable in the home environment; care providers as motivators; care partner decreases loneliness/isolation | Describe the scheme and content of ESD and continued rehabilitation strategy as evolved in the research program at Huddinge University Hospital for patient with moderate neurologic impairments. | OT, PT, SP provided in home for an average of 14 wk (range: 4–29 wk), patients received an average of 15 h of therapy (range: 2–44 h); part of RCT? = no |

Abbreviations: OT, occupational therapy; PT, physical therapy; RCT, randomized controlled trial; SP, speech pathology.

Table 2
Critical Appraisal Skills Programme: quality assessment tool

	Taule and Raheim,[6] 2014	Chouliara et al,[11] 2014	Collins et al,[8] 2016	Cobley et al,[12] 2013	Taule et al,[7] 2015	Lou et al,[10] 2017	von Koch et al,[9] 2000
Was there a clear statement of the aims of the research?	Yes	Yes	Yes	Yes	Yes	Yes	Yes
Is a qualitative methodology appropriate?	Yes	Yes	Yes	Yes	Yes	Yes	Yes
Was the research design appropriate to address the aims of the research?	Yes	Cannot tell	Yes	Yes	Yes	Yes	No
Was the recruitment strategy appropriate to the aims of the research?	Yes	Yes	No	Yes	Yes	Yes	Yes
Were the data collected in a way that addressed the research issue?	No	No	No	Yes	No	Yes	Yes
Has the relationship between researcher and participants been adequately considered?	Yes	No	No	No	Yes	No	No
Have ethical issues been taken into consideration?	Yes	Cannot tell	Yes	Yes	Yes	Yes	Yes
Were the data analysis sufficiently rigorous?	Yes	Yes	Yes	Yes	Yes	Yes	Yes
Is there a clear statement of findings?	Yes	Yes	Yes	Yes	Yes	Yes	Yes
How valuable is the research?	Yes	Yes	Yes	Yes	Yes	Yes	Yes

patient-provider relationship. The second theme was experiences of logistical components of ESD and included 2 subthemes: (1) the experience and understanding of the ESD process and (2) home environment—the space where the rehabilitation intervention took place.

THE PSYCHOSOCIAL ASPECTS OF EARLY SUPPORTED DISCHARGE
The Emotional Experience: Hope, Desire, and Sense of Loss

Four of the 6 studies emphasized the emotional experience of ESD as a main theme.[6–8,10] In 2 of these studies, the patients unanimously agreed they felt ready to discharge from a specialized stroke unit and (See Norma D. McNair's article, "The Projected Transition Trajectory for Survivors and Carers of Patients Who Have Had a Stroke," in this issue).[8,10] Discharge was viewed as a major milestone in the rehabilitation process and symbolized to the patients that their health care providers were confident they were ready to integrate back into the community. Despite feelings of anxiety and uncertainty about experiencing their homes with a changed functional capacity, patients reported a yearning to return home.[8,10]

Patients in 3 of the studies emphasized the importance of specific inherent characteristics of an ideal ESD patient candidate, such as optimism and determination.[6–8,10]

And although patients worried about the future, their functioning ability, and the risk of another stroke,[7,8,10] 2 of the 3 studies reported patients were generally optimistic and had hope for the future.[8,10] Patients and carers expressed hope for a full recovery and a return to activities that brought them pleasure and satisfaction.[10] One patient said:

> I think an awful lot of it has to do with the patient. The type of patient that you have. You either have somebody who's helpless and not strong enough to face it...but...if you can make yourself, do it! You have to make yourself; same as you have to make yourself get up and walk.[8]

Taule and colleges[7] reported that patients viewed hope as the driving force behind their recovery. Yet patients in this study found it difficult to find hope at times. Changes in physical and cognitive abilities effected self-esteem, and they struggled to make sense of the confusing split between the emotional drive to complete a task and a body unable to fulfill the desire.[7] Patients reported that pain, fatigue, uncertainty about health, inability to return to driving and work, and loss of independence contributed to an underlying sadness and a sense of loss of freedom. Patients experienced changes in relationships and reported that less contact with friends and colleagues resulted in feelings of aloneness.[7] A grandfather says of his relationship with his grandson:

> He withdraws a bit. And he, yes, he does not express it so explicitly (crying), but I do not have the same contact with him, like before. And he knows I can't (crying), eh (swallowing), that grandfather can't take him out fishing (voice cracking) fishing again.[6]

Relationships: Patients, Carers, and Providers

Five of the 6 studies reported on the patient-provider relationship.[7–10,12] Disciplines represented on the ESD provider team vary by program but teams are composed of physical therapists, occupational therapists, and speech therapists, and nurses. Patients, carers, and providers agreed that the patient-provider relationship was richer and more rewarding than it would have been in the hospital.[8–10] Patients believed they established a close relationship with their provider because the provider was incorporated into their personal life and had an intimate understanding of the their roles and routines within the context of daily life in the home.[7–10,12] Taule and colleagues[7] found that patients were heavily influenced by their provider's attitude and communication style. Providers who conveyed empathy and listened to patient concerns resulted in patients feeling empowered and hopeful about recovery. Providers cultivated trusting relationships with patients when they provided the honest balance between optimism and realism. This balance fostered hope for the future and also a sense of what to expect and how to compensate for long-term deficits.

Lou and colleagues[10] reported that both patients and carers believed that participating in rehabilitation at home promoted an open and equitable relationship between the patient, the provider, and the carer. Patients reported that relationships evolved over time. Initially providers were viewed as strangers, provoking patient anxiety but, over time, were viewed as knowledgeable friends whose visits were highly valued.[8] Patients reported that they missed the providers and the social aspect of therapy when ESD concluded.[10] One patient's perspective was:

> It's just more relaxed...Like, at the hospital I sit in the chair, right? At the patient side of the table. But at home it's different. It's my home ground so the roles are a bit different. She's the visitor. That puts me in more control, in a way.[10]

Carers reported appreciation for providers in the home, perceiving them as implementers of structure and, at times, firmness with the patients. Carers believed that had they interacted with patients with the same dynamics, it may have been interpreted negatively and jeopardized the relationship over time.[10] Carers also viewed the time patients spent with the providers as a time of respite, a time to engage in their own valued activities. A few believed, however, that the therapeutic interventions were not long enough and felt housebound when providers were present. Carers in Cobley and colleagues'[12] study reported feeling physically drained by their new role and ill informed about what to expect and how best to care for their loved ones. They felt unsupported by providers, reporting a lack of education, training, and information.

von Koch and colleagues[9] reported that the ESD providers emphasized their role as listeners. Providers spent a substantial amount of time in dialogue with the patients and believed that communication was an essential ingredient of a productive partnership. They also believed it was important to allow the patient to guide the therapy sessions. One provider stated:

> In the hospital, this big institution where you are an authority in a white coat, the patient submits himself to you and wants you to help him and make him well. But at home, I think it's more like you discuss the patient's problems and co-operate with him to find solutions.[9]

THE LOGISTICAL COMPONENTS OF EARLY SUPPORTED DISCHARGE

All the studies reported on aspects of the ESD process, including logistical components, such as patient eligibility criteria, the nature of the intervention provided (frequency, intensity, and content), communication for care-level transition, and consideration of who provides the care and how. The ESD process varied substantially from study to study and took place in the context of a variety of medical systems.

Provider-to-Provider Communication

Three studies highlighted the importance of communication between providers in planning the transitions and treatment intervention.[6,8,11] Communication between members of the treatment team was a crucial component for continuity of care and reduction of duplicated of services. Providers also reported that communication between acute care staff and ESD providers was key to identifying patients who were deemed appropriate for ESD services.[10] von Koch and colleagues[9] reported that ESD providers were enthusiastic about the use of weekly team meetings to foster communication, where providers assisted, supported, taught, and learned from each other. Several providers identified lack of communication between disciplines as contributing to duplication of services. They believed that a data-sharing system would eliminate this problem.[11] Communication with service extenders also was viewed as important. In the study by Chouliara and colleagues,[11] rehabilitation assistance was used to deliver treatment to less complicated patients. Assistants were a key component of the sustainability of ESD services. This model, however, required clear communications between personnel.[10]

Transitions: Hospital to Home to Community

Five studies discussed the process of transitioning home. The studies suggested that although patients were satisfied with the treatment provided, they lacked an understanding of the process and were, at times, disappointed when treatment ended without full recovery.[4,5,7,9,10] Cobley and colleagues[12] reported patients found the transition from hospital to home to be seamless, with ESD initial visits occurring within 24 hours of discharge. Overall, patients were satisfied with therapy, which included up to 4 visits per day, 7 days a week, for 6 weeks. These patients were dissatisfied, however, with the transition from ESD intervention to community services, reporting that treatment seemed to end abruptly at 6 weeks regardless of the progress made, and the transition to community-based services was not well managed. Some patients in Taule and colleagues'[7] study expressed a similar dissatisfaction with transitioning from ESD services to community-based services, reporting they felt betrayed by trusted providers when valuable rehabilitation time was lost due to paperwork logistics required for transition of care.

In Collins and colleagues' study,[8] patients reported limited understanding of ESD. The initial decision to participate in ESD was made early after diagnosis during a time of uncertainty and confusion. A patient was asked about his understanding of the ESD process, stating:

To be quite honest with you, I don't know how to describe it...they [staff in the hospital] told me I'd get home; they told me about this...then just in a couple of days I got home here.[8]

In Lou and colleagues' study[10] in the Central Denmark Region patients received 1 to 4 visits from an ESD provider and, if care was required beyond 4 visits, patients were referred to community-based health services. Two patients were unsatisfied with ESD and community services. They reported that they were eager to return work and believed that the interventions were focused on basic activities of daily living (ADLs) and did not address return-to-work needs.

Environment

Five of the 6 studies reported on the experience of rehabilitation in the home environment.[8–12] Participants in all 5 studies conveyed the home as ideal for rehabilitation after mild to moderate stroke. Patients reported they felt empowered because, within their own space, they could guide the intervention. They had a sense of control in a familiar space that they may not have experienced in a hospital setting.[8,10] They also reported that interventions in the home were tailored to their needs in a way that was not possible in the hospital.[8,12] One patient reported:

Walking up and down the gym in the hospital is great but it's not walking to the different levels of my floor in my home.[8]

Patients described the hospital environment as busy and impersonal, a place where time and space are structured around hospital practices and routines that may not be the practices and routines of the individual patients.[10] Some patients reported they felt secure about participating in an ESD program because they shared a home with their carer. They expressed it would be much more daunting to participate in ESD if they were discharged home to live alone.[10] Home served as a laboratory where patients could test their abilities, evaluate their capacity, brainstorm, practice, and problem-solve in their natural environment.[9,10] But, for some, the home environment emphasized deficits and limitations, a daily reminder of the activities in which they could no longer participate independently.[10]

Providers reported that home provided an ecologically valid assessment of ADL deficits, making it more feasible to tailor treatment sessions to a patient's specific needs.[9,11] One provider stated:

It is less about a body in a bed that needs a bit of fixing; to me, it feels more of a holistic service; just being in peoples' houses, seeing what problems they actually have and adapting the service around that.[11]

Providers found they were able to provide a more patient-centered intervention in the home compared with in the hospital, and over time they adopted a new treatment philosophy requiring their patients to take an active role in treatment and problem-solving strategizing.[9]

Eligibility criteria and community resources were identified as important for ESD. Providers in Chouliara and colleagues'[11] study were generally positive about their hospital's eligibility criteria for ESD enrollment. Some, however, felt the lack of community services for patients with severe deficits resulted in some patients inappropriately enrolled in the ESD program. Providers felt they were over-extended and unable to provide appropriate care to patients with severe deficits or unsuitable home conditions.

DISCUSSION

This review synthesizes the overall patient, carer, and provider experience of myriad ESD service models delivered in several countries within a variety of medical systems. ESD intervention is not a standardized approach; programs vary greatly in organization, content, length, and frequency of visits.[9,13,14] Programs in this review ranged from 1 visit to 4 visits to up to 29 weeks of therapeutic intervention. Three of the studies did not provide a description of the program.[7,8,12] The remaining 3 described the ESD program as multidisciplinary (occupational therapy, physical therapy, speech therapy, and nursing). One intervention was daily for up to 7 days a week,[11] another was 1 to 2 visits per week,[9] and the third was 1 to 4 visits total.[10] The content and length of each visit were not specified, although 1 study reported that patients received an average total of 15 hours of therapy.[9] None of the studies described the transition process from hospital to ESD services or ESD to community-based services, and the nature of community-based services beyond ESD was not defined.

A recent systematic review established determinants influencing ESD implementation and outcomes and concluded there are specific attributes rendering ESD programs a success. Program success was defined as "superior compared to alternative interventions."[15] The attributes can be categorized into the same 2 main themes revealed in this qualitative review (1) psychosocial aspects—personal needs, level of motivation, values, goals, skills, learning style, and social network and (2) logistical components of the program—compatibility of the program with the values of the patient or the provider, complexity of the program, and aspects of the organization, such as size, structure, and available expertise.[15,16]

The quantitative review found that a collaborative approach between provider and patient resulted in smoother transitions and increased patient involvement and application of problem-solving skills.[15] Degree of collaboration was determined not only by patient willingness but also by the values and beliefs of the provider.[17] In this qualitative review, patients and providers seemed to take the concept of collaboration a step further, describing the patient-provider relationship as a crucial aspect of the experience of ESD, one that influences multiple dimensions of recovery and overall satisfaction with the ESD program.

Another main determinant of successful ESD programs is care coordination. Successful ESD programs appoint case managers or multidisciplinary teams to coordinate patient care from hospital discharge to ESD discharge.[18] A stepwise approach is recommended where patients and carers are weaned from therapeutic intervention, interacting with a provider less and less frequently until they are capable of functioning on their own.[19] This theme was also prominent in this qualitative review. Patients expressed that times of transition of care level are when they feel most vulnerable.[7] They reported mixed experiences of transition; some reported seamless transitions cultivating trust in the program whereas others reported that an unstable transition resulted in unnecessary anxiety and the loss of therapeutic intervention during a critical time of recovery. The importance of communication also was emphasized. Care coordination requires clear and frequent communication between care managers, providers, carers, patients, and community-based services. Providers stressed the crucial role of provider-to-provider communication to prevent duplication of services and promote a clear clinical picture of the patient and their home situation.

The review of determinants of a successful ESD program defines ESD simply as "...a shift of rehabilitation services from clinical to home setting with no change in the content of rehabilitation...mainly [a] restructuring of the timing and location of the service delivery."[15] Yet, the findings from this qualitative review suggest the experience of ESD is more than this. Participating in early intervention in the home rather than a hospital may provide a more ecologically valid assessment of patient independence and may increase motivation and determination as patients return to familiar roles and routines. Patients and carers valued the familiarity of their own space; they felt empowered and more in control of the intervention. The home environment encouraged problem solving and enriched the patient-provider relationship because providers were integrated into the intimate daily lives of the patients. Providers found the home cultivated patient-centered treatment and served as a true measure of ADL independence. Patients, carers, and providers found meaning in the ESD intervention and in the relationships formulated during the process.

Overall, patients, carers, and providers reported a positive experience of ESD. Yet, no study has explored a qualitative comparison between those who experience ESD and those who experience the conventional rehabilitation process. Piccenna and colleagues[20] conducted a review of qualitative studies examining the patient and carer experience of the transition from hospital to home during conventional rehabilitation after acquired brain injury. The review included 9 studies of moderate quality and concluded that patients and carers were generally unsatisfied with their transition from hospital to home. They reported lack of communication, lack of information regarding the disease process and how to manage a chronic condition, and poor community-based support as the major deficiencies of the process. These areas of concern were similarly expressed among those who experienced the ESD process. Despite evidence suggesting ESD is equally or more effective than center-based rehabilitation in terms of hospital readmission, ADL outcomes, and social functioning,[18] patients and carers who experienced ESD reported the same program deficits as patients and carers who experienced conventional rehabilitation. This suggests a need for more research into implementation of self-management and self-management support throughout the rehabilitation process for neurorehabilitation patients and their carers.

Patients with stroke and their carers reported a lack of educational information and problem-solving skills necessary to solve problems as they arose once discharged home.[21–23] Individuals who believe in their ability to self-manage their care are more likely to employ and sustain actions promoting functional independence after stroke.[24] The core tenets of self-management, as described by Lorig and Holman, include (1) autonomy and control, (2) ability and responsibility, (3) a problem-based approach revolving around perceived needs, (4) tailoring to readiness to learn/change and beliefs about health, and (5) the realization that self-management always occurs through active management or through chosen nonmanagement.[25] Problem-solving theories emphasize how critical problem solving is for effective self-management.[26] Recent evidence suggests formal training using a problem-solving approach equips patients and carers with abilities to translate education and training into effective action[27] and instills the necessary skills to manage problems or barriers that arise after hospital discharge and beyond.[28]

Based on the findings of this qualitative review combined with insight gleaned from the systematic review of established determinants influencing ESD implementation[15] and the qualitative review of patient, carer, and provider experiences of traditional transition from inpatient rehabilitation to the community.[20] Future research is warranted in several areas, such as size, structure, dosing, and timing of home-based intervention. Currently, there is no standardization of ESD implementation. Research is also needed to better understand the psychosocial needs of patients with stroke and their carers at vulnerable times of transition between levels of care. Finally, more research is warranted in the area of patient and carer self-management strategy training in order to best prepare patients and carers for new roles and routines after stroke.

LIMITATIONS

This qualitative review included only studies published in English in peer-reviewed journals. This criteria may have excluded studies providing additional insight into the experience of ESD. Also, the CASP, used to evaluate the quality of the studies included, may not be a robust appraisal tool. There currently is no consensus regarding qualitative appraisal tools within qualitative research.

SUMMARY

Patients, carers, and providers generally had a positive view of the ESD experience, although patient and carers interviewed several months after the experience seemed to harbor more anxiety and concern for the future. Those who experienced ESD emphasized psychosocial aspects of program—development of the patient-provider relationship, the comforts of returning to a daily routine in a familiar space, and the ability to tailor treatment to meet patient-oriented goals. Patients, carers, and providers all stressed the importance of systematic communication between all parties involved in the process. ESD outcomes research around the world suggests ESD may be a viable rehabilitation option for patients with mild to moderate stroke.[29] Yet, this research and ESD program development remains in its infancy. More research regarding ESD outcomes and patient, carer, and provider experiences is warranted to best meet the needs of patients with stroke and their family members.

REFERENCES

1. Ellis-Hill C, Robison J, Wiles R, et al. Going home to get on with life: patients and carers experiences of being discharged from hospital following a stroke. Disabil Rehabil 2009;31(2):61–72.
2. Flick U, Von Kardorff E, Steinke I. What is qualitative research? An introduction to the field. *A companion to qualitative research*. In:2004:3–11.
3. Critical Appraisal Skills Programme (CASP). Qualitative research checklist. Oxford: Better Value Healthcare LTD; 1993. Available at: https://casp-uk.net/casp-tools-checklists/.

4. Booth A. Supplementary guidance for inclusion of qualitative research in Cochrane systematic reviews of intervention. Cochrane Collaboration Qualitative Methods Group; 2011. Version 1.
5. Krueger R, Casey M. Focus groups: a practical guide for applied research. 5th edition. Thousand Oaks (CA): SAGE Publications Inc; 2014.
6. Taule T, Raheim M. Life changed existentially: a qualitative study of experiences at 6-8 months after mild stroke. Disabil Rehabil 2014;36(25):2107–19.
7. Taule T, Strand LI, Skouen JS, et al. Striving for a life worth living: stroke survivors' experiences of home rehabilitation. Scand J Caring Sci 2015;29(4):651–61.
8. Collins G, Breen C, Walsh T, et al. An exploration of the experience of early supported discharge from the perspective of stroke survivors. Int J Ther Rehabil 2016;23:207–14.
9. von Koch L, Holmqvist LW, Wottrich AW, et al. Rehabilitation at home after stroke: a descriptive study of an individualized intervention. Clin Rehabil 2000;14(6):574–83.
10. Lou S, Carstensen K, Moldrup M, et al. Early supported discharge following mild stroke: a qualitative study of patients' and their partners' experiences of rehabilitation at home. Scand J Caring Sci 2017;31(2):302–11.
11. Chouliara N, Fisher RJ, Kerr M, et al. Implementing evidence-based stroke early supported discharge services: a qualitative study of challenges, facilitators and impact. Clin Rehabil 2014;28(4):370–7.
12. Cobley CS, Fisher RJ, Chouliara N, et al. A qualitative study exploring patients' and carers' experiences of Early Supported Discharge services after stroke. Clin Rehabil 2013;27(8):750–7.
13. Cunliffe AL, Gladman JR, Husbands SL, et al. Sooner and healthier: a randomised controlled trial and interview study of an early discharge rehabilitation service for older people. Age Ageing 2004;33(3):246–52.
14. Geddes JM, Chamberlain MA. Home-based rehabilitation for people with stroke: a comparative study of six community services providing co-ordinated, multidisciplinary treatment. Clin Rehabil 2001;15(6):589–99.
15. Siemonsma P, Dopp C, Alpay L, et al. Determinants influencing the implementation of home-based stroke rehabilitation: a systematic review. Disabil Rehabil 2014;36(24):2019–30.
16. Fleuren M, Wiefferink K, Paulussen T. Determinants of innovation within health care organizations: literature review and Delphi study. Int J Qual Health Care 2004;16(2):107–23.
17. Rogers EM. Diffusions of innovations. 5th edition. New York: Free Press; 2003.
18. Langhorne P, Holmqvist LW. Early supported discharge after stroke. J Rehabil Med 2007;39(2):103–8.
19. Larsen T, Olsen TS, Sorensen J. Early home-supported discharge of stroke patients: a health technology assessment. Int J Technol Assess Health Care 2006;22(3):313–20.
20. Piccenna L, Lannin NA, Gruen R, et al. The experience of discharge for patients with an acquired brain injury from the inpatient to the community setting: a qualitative review. Brain Inj 2016;30(3):241–51.
21. Chen L, Xiao LD, De Bellis A. First-time stroke survivors and caregivers' perceptions of being engaged in rehabilitation. J Adv Nurs 2016;72(1):73–84.
22. Magasi S, Durkin E, Wolf MS, et al. Rehabilitation consumers' use and understanding of quality information: a health literacy perspective. Arch Phys Med Rehabil 2009;90(2):206–12.

23. Laver K, Halbert J, Stewart M, et al. Patient readiness and ability to set recovery goals during the first 6 months after stroke. J Allied Health 2010;39(4):e149–54.
24. Jones F, Riazi A. Self-efficacy and self-management after stroke: a systematic review. Disabil Rehabil 2011;33(10):797–810.
25. Lorig KR, Holman H. Self-management education: history, definition, outcomes, and mechanisms. Ann Behav Med 2003;26(1):1–7.
26. D'Zurilla TJ, Nezu AM, Maydeu-Olivares A. Social problem solving: theory and assessment 2004.
27. Portillo MC, Corchon S, Lopez-Dicastillo O, et al. Evaluation of a nurse-led social rehabilitation programme for neurological patients and carers: an action research study. Int J Nurs Stud 2009;46(2):204–19.
28. Malouff JM, Thorsteinsson EB, Schutte NS. The efficacy of problem solving therapy in reducing mental and physical health problems: a meta-analysis. Clin Psychol Rev 2007;27(1):46–57.
29. Langhorne P, Baylan S. Early supported discharge services for people with acute stroke. Cochrane Database Syst Rev 2017;(7):CD000443.

The Hospital to Home Transition Following Acute Stroke

DaiWai M. Olson, PhD, RN, CCRN, FNCS[a],*,
Shannon B. Juengst, PhD, CRC[b]

KEYWORDS

- Stroke • Neuroscience nursing • Transitional care • Patient transfer

KEY POINTS

- Early supported discharge is the most widely studied intervention, and currently represents the most evidence-based intervention, for hospital to home transitions after acute stroke.
- The use of usual care as a comparator for interventional studies significantly limits the generalizability of results for studies examining transition of care interventions.
- All of the studies included in this update assessed outcomes between 3 and 12 months. However, there was no consistency in selecting outcome measures.

INTRODUCTION

Morbidity and mortality rates attributed to the immediate effects of acute stroke have steadily declined, resulting in more patients discharged home after being hospitalized for stroke. However, best practice for optimizing the transition of care (TOC) from hospital to home is poorly understood. The most significant body of work providing insight into stroke TOC was a 2011 report, funded by the Agency for Healthcare Research and Quality (AHRQ),[1] and subsequent summary manuscript of the systematic review including myocardial infarction (MI) and ischemic stroke.[2] Before March 2012, only 44 published manuscripts discussed stroke TOC research. Four types of intervention emerged as representative of evidence-based mechanisms to improve TOC from hospital to home after stroke: (1) hospital-initiated support, (2) patient and family education, (3) community-based support, and (4) chronic disease management. Building on

Disclosure Statement: Dr D.M. Olson declares that he is the editor for the Journal of Neuroscience Nursing. Dr S.B. Juengst declares no conflicts of interest.
[a] Neurology and Neurotherapeutics, University of Texas Southwestern, 5323 Harry Hines Boulevard, Dallas, TX 75390-8897, USA; [b] Physical Medicine and Rehabilitation, University of Texas Southwestern, 5323 Harry Hines Boulevard, Dallas, TX 75390-9055, USA
* Corresponding author.
E-mail address: DaiWai.Olson@UTSouthwestern.edu

that work, this article provides a comprehensive update on stroke TOC including relevant research published in the intervening decade, up to June 2018, and to provide practice and research recommendations.

BACKGROUND AND SIGNIFICANCE

Stroke is associated with significant morbidity and mortality.[3] Worldwide, roughly 15 million stroke events occur yearly, with incidence rates ranging from 76 to 119 per 100,000 per year depending on country.[4,5] The incidence is higher in men versus women and most strokes are ischemic (vs hemorrhagic). The evolution of stroke care over the past 50 years created new challenges and new opportunities.[6] Advances in early stroke treatment increased the number of stroke patients discharged home (vs to inpatient rehabilitation facility, skilled nursing facility, or long-term acute care center). In large part because of global efforts to promote early intervention, the use of thrombolytic medications, such as alteplase or tenecteplase, has increased.[7] More recently, mechanical thrombectomy procedures extended the treatment window for ischemic stroke.[8] Hemorrhagic stroke (intracranial hemorrhage [ICH] and subarachnoid hemorrhage) treatment algorithms have also reduced morbidity and mortality.[9]

It is not surprising that increased stroke survival subsequently increased the number of stroke survivors going home after discharge. What is surprising is the failure of the medical community to keep pace with an ever-increasing demand for interventions that improve long-term success by facilitating TOC for stroke. The successful implementation of stroke programs and protocols, although hypothesized to reduce the burden of stroke,[9] may actually increase the global burden of this disease. The last summary of evidence for TOC was in 2011[1] and included stroke and MI. Although stroke and MI are cardiovascular events, including both disease states in a single report was a major criticism from public comment on the report.[10]

The AHRQ report on TOC supports implementation of hospital-initiated interventions. In particular, early supported discharge (ESD) has promise to improve TOC following acute stroke.[1] ESD interventions are those in which a patient is discharged earlier than normal and receives additional support beyond the standard-of-care; moreover, the support intervention must begin before hospital discharge.[11] The AHRQ report noted limitations including small sample size, heterogeneity of outcome measures across studies, and limited discussion of control or baseline conditions. Despite anecdotal evidence (platform presentations at nursing conferences) of an increase in ESD interventions, there has been no formal appraisal of TOC for acute stroke since 2011. Therefore, this article fills the gap in summary literature in the intervening decade and to provide practice and research recommendations.

Search Strategy

The primary aim being to update the literature, the first step was to examine literature published after the 2011 summary. A university librarian performed a comprehensive search to find literature published in PubMed, CINAHL, and Embase using established criteria from previous TOC literature.[1,2] The PubMed search used the Mesh terms (stroke, critical pathways, physical therapy modalities, case management, rehabilitation, continuity of care, patient discharge, patient transfer, postacute care, skilled nursing facilities, assisted living facilities, transfer of care, transition, postdischarge, posthospital, subacute care, referral, and continuity). This search was limited to include all forms of trials (randomized, clinical, crossover, meta-analyses, case-control, cohort, and follow-up), published after January 1, 2012. This search was replicated in CINAHL and Embase with appropriate customizations for each library database. Results from each database were compiled into a single EndNote library and duplicates removed.

FINDINGS

The search revealed 4625 potentially relevant articles. After title and abstract review, 43 articles remained and were subjected to full read by both authors. Of these, 34 were excluded for: not studying transition from hospital to home (24), only including qualitative data (four), no intervention studied (four), review article (one), and duplicate publication (one). The nine remaining articles were included in this analysis (**Table 1**).[12–20]

In 2013, Hohmann and colleagues[14] examined 3-month medication adherence in 310 patients (155 control subjects, 155 intervention) with stroke or transient ischemic attack (TIA) taking at least two medications. This nonrandomized trial studied an intervention focusing on the primary care physician. The control group received a discharge letter to share with their primary care physician that detailed their diagnosis, test results, and medications. The intervention was delivered by a clinical pharmacist and included patient education. By contrast, the intervention group's discharge letter included detailed information for all medication changes from admission to discharge and reasons for changes, with a focus on reasons for clinical decisions about antithrombotic drugs and adding simvastatin. Overall, perfect adherence to the medication regimen was 90.9% in the intervention group, indicating the intervention resulted in better adherence than the control group (83.3% adherence; $P = .01$).

In a planned secondary analysis of 61 patients, Brown and colleagues[20] examined participation in an aerobic fitness program (n = 35) of three sessions per week for 10 to 30 minutes per session before discharge. Outcomes were compared with nonparticipation (n = 26). The intervention group also received three postdischarge follow-up telephone calls in the first 6 months after discharge to assess physical activity. Although participants in the intervention group were discharged earlier than nonparticipants, potentially because of factors associated with initial nonparticipation, they were neither more nor less likely to participate in an exercise program after discharge.[20]

In 2014, Nayeri and colleagues[15] examined 60 Iranian dyads; 60 patients with first ischemic stroke and their 60 care partners. Dyads were enrolled within 48 hours of stroke and followed for 2 months. The intervention group received an individualized family-centered care program consisting of needs assessment, tailored education, follow-up postdischarge via telephone, and assistance coordinating health care referrals. The control group received usual care (defined only as "the routing care provided by the hospital").[15] The intervention was associated with fewer readmissions, fewer instances of pneumonia/respiratory infection or bedsores after discharge, and higher therapeutic adherence scores.

In 2016, Bodechtel and colleagues[12] study compared 45 patients with stroke receiving a standardized post-stroke pathway intervention, primarily providing and reinforcing stroke-based education, with 45 matched control subjects receiving usual care. The post-stroke pathway intervention began at admission and included a planned 1-week in-home follow-up; planned interval telephone follow-up at 3, 6, and 9 months; and an in-home follow-up at 1 year. At 1-year post-stroke, patients in the intervention group achieved blood pressure, cholesterol, and body mass index goals; were more functionally independent; and reported higher quality of life than control subjects.

A study out of Copenhagen, also in 2016,[17] used a multidisciplinary approach to coordinate home-based rehabilitation after discharge for 31 patients with stroke, versus

Table 1
Articles retained in the 2019 update

First Author, Year	Sample (Size)	Intervention	Comparator	Primary Outcome	Timing
Hohmann et al,[14] 2013	AIS, TIA (310)	CBS: enhanced medication communication for primary providers	Standard communication	Medication adherence	3 mo
Brown et al,[20] 2014	Stroke (61)	ESD: physical therapy exercise program	Usual care	Postdischarge physical activity	6 mo
Nayeri et al,[15] 2014	AIS, CP (60 dyads)	ESD: 4-step family-centered care program	Usual care	Adherence to therapeutic regimen	2 mo
Bodechtel et al,[12] 2016	AIS, TIA (90)	PFE: planned interval teaching and medication coaching	Matched control subjects Usual care	Risk factor reduction	12 mo
Rasmussen et al,[17] 2016	Stroke (61)	ESD: coordinated home-based rehabilitation	Usual care	Physical, cognitive, and quality of life measures	3 mo
Santana et al,[18] 2017	AIS, TIA, ICH (190)	ESD: Early home-supported discharge homecare team	Usual care	FIM scores	2 mo and 6 mo
Olaiya et al,[16] 2017	Stroke, TIA (563)	CDM: chronic disease management and stroke education	Usual care	Framingham Risk Score	12 mo
Vanacker et al,[19] 2017	AIS (255)	ESD: stroke coach	Usual care	Medication adherence	3 mo
Deen et al,[13] 2018	Stroke (100)	CBS: stroke nurse navigator program	Historical cohort	Adherence to plan of care	12 mo

Abbreviations: AIS, acute ischemic stroke; CBS, community-based support; CDM, chronic disease management; CP, care partner/caregiver; FIM, functional independence measure; PFE, patient family education; Stroke, not otherwise specified; TIA, transient ischemic attack.

30 patients receiving usual care, and compared disability, motor, and cognitive function, and quality of life at 90 days post-stroke. In contrast to other studies, the length of stay was longer (but not statistically different) for the intervention versus control patients. There was, however, greater improvement in modified Rankin scale scores and motor assessment scale scores in the intervention group, and they also reported significantly higher quality of life, compared with control subjects, at 90-days post stroke.

The focus on ESD was again evident in Santana and colleagues'[18] 2017 Portuguese study. They randomized 190 patients with stroke to early home-supported discharge (EHSD) versus usual care. EHSD began during the patient's stroke unit stay. Both the

EHSD and control (usual care) subjects received rehabilitation as standard of care. The EHSD patients discharged home received an individual rehabilitation plan, including aids and modifications as feasible. Seventeen patients in the EHSD group went to inpatient rehabilitation from the stroke unit, after which contact with the EHSD case manager was re-established before discharge home. Patients in the usual care group also had a case manager who provided only basic information about services available in the community. The authors found no differences in functional independence measure scores at 6 months, although there was some indication that EHSD may result in greater improvement than usual care among those with particularly low (<60) functional independence measure scores.

Two other studies published in 2017 focused on a stroke nurse navigator approach and stroke coach program.[16,19] Olaiya and colleagues[16] conducted a multicenter, cluster-randomized controlled trial of usual care (n = 280) versus an individualized chronic disease management plan developed through a nurse-led shared team approach (n = 283) to improve cardiovascular risk management after discharge. The chronic disease management plan was developed during the inpatient stay by a nurse, in consultation with stroke specialists, and then the nurse made a home visit postdischarge to provide education tailored to the individual's risk factors. The authors found no differences between groups for any outcome measure, including Framingham Risk Score or blood pressure.

Vanacker and colleagues[19] assessed the efficacy of a stroke coach program delivered to 74 individuals with ischemic stroke, compared with historical control subjects (n = 79). The stroke coach, who was an experienced stroke nurse, contacted patients twice before discharge and then up to five times postdischarge to discuss managing risk factors and to review medications. Compared with the control group (usual care), the stroke coach group had 1-day shorter length of in-hospital stay. Stroke coach participants had significantly better adherence at 3 months post-stroke to all medications, save for antiglycemic drugs. Few participants were able to be contacted via telephone postdischarge, but most (73%) were routinely seen at 1-, 3-, and 6-month ambulatory visits.

Only one paper was published in 2018, discussing research from a TOC stroke study[13]; this explored a stroke nurse navigation program (SNNP). Although stroke is inadequately defined, this extensive analysis examines pre-post data before and after implementation of a detailed SNNP program that began during hospitalization, included postdischarge follow-up, and contact with patients who experienced rehospitalization. The primary analysis explores the impact of SNNP on 100 patients during the first year after acute ischemic stroke (AIS). SNNP was associated with higher adherence to medication and follow-up appointments and fewer emergency department visits. The authors noted that during the first year after discharge, AIS patients had a trend toward lower quality of life compared with baseline. Notably, the authors provide insight toward TOC areas ripe for outcomes research, including medication adherence, health care follow-up, readmission (including emergency department visit), quality of life, and ability to complete activities of daily living.

Populations Included

Five studies included AIS. Of these, 2 included TIA, 1 included TIA and ICH, and one included care partners. Four studies enrolled patients with unspecified stroke type (ie, AIS, TIA, ICH, or subarachnoid hemorrhage). Of these, one did note including TIA, and it is reasonable to assume that this was a study of AIS and TIA. Although 2 studies included only AIS (with/without care partner), no studies focused only on TOC for hemorrhagic stroke or only on TIA. All of the studies included a broad age range of adults;

none focused on narrow age ranges, such as young adult (author note: pediatric stroke was a search exclusion criterion). No studies targeted enrollment to only 1 sex, and no studies documented or cited support that TOC experiences differ for males versus females.

Interventions

The interventions across the 9 reviewed studies varied considerably. Some focused narrowly on a particular outcome, including one detailed letter about medications to improve medication adherence and one inpatient fitness program to improve postdischarge physical activity. Others were broader, case management-based interventions, including a stroke coach program, EHSD, a family-centered care program, 1 stroke nurse navigator, 1 nurse-led chronic disease management program, and 2 more rehabilitation-focused program (home-based rehabilitation during hospitalization and a functionally oriented standardized post-stroke pathway). As noted in the 2011 AHRQ report,[21] the most common comparator was usual care.

Outcomes

Although outcome measures varied broadly in construct and timing, the primary outcomes were essentially adherence, physical function, or risk reduction. Primary outcomes were adherence (4 studies),[13–15,19] medication adherence (2 studies),[14,19] and plan of care adherence (2 studies).[13,15] Adherence outcomes were assessed at 2, 6, and 12 months. Three studies' primary outcome was physical function, measured at 90 days, 2 months, and 6 months postdischarge.[17,18,20] The 2 remaining studies focused on risk factor reduction 12 months postdischarge.[12,16] Three studies examined length of stay and found shorter, but not statistically significantly different, length of stay was associated with the intervention.[17,18,20]

DISCUSSION

The 9 new studies[12–20] included in this report have remarkable similarities and deficiencies with the previous 41 stroke articles[22–63] from the 2011 AHRQ report.[21] Regarding TOC from hospital to home after acute stroke, there is still only limited evidence available to support any specific intervention, outcome, or time point at which to measure outcomes. This finding echoes sentiments from the 2016 Canadian TOC guidelines, which specifically state that recommendations "are not supported by randomized controlled trials or meta-analyses."[64]

Population

The generalist approach to population and sampling continues to pervade TOC stroke literature. This may signal that TOC research is still in its infancy, or it may reflect investigator naiveté in the assumption that TOC is similar across all diagnoses and patient subtypes.[65] Including 2 major cardiovascular events in the same report was a major shortcoming of the AHRQ report.[10] Not only should stroke be separate from other diseases, but a growing body of evidence suggests that a single category for stroke may be too broad. The needs and trajectories of patients recovering from ischemic stroke are different than patients recovering from hemorrhagic stroke, and recovery trajectory varies by patient age, sex, stroke severity, and available resources.[66–68] In tandem to the personalized medicine campaigns, there is a need to define which subsets of the population are most likely to benefit from the various TOC interventions.

It is encouraging to see progression, especially in nursing literature, toward including care partners and exploring the contributions of dyadic relationships. The term care partner reflects an extended member of the stroke patient's family (friends) who may not provide direct assistance, but is contributing to the well-being of and sharing the lived experience with the patient.[69] The term caregiver should be reserved for persons whose primary role is specifically providing/giving health care assistance.[70]

Intervention

The 4 primary intervention categories identified in 2012 were: (1) hospital-initiated discharge support, (2) patient-family education, (3) community based support, and (4) chronic disease management.[21] Five of the nine newly identified interventions could be classified as ESD and would fall into the category of hospital-initiated discharge support.[15,17–20] Two of the newer studies provided new evidence in favor of community-based support interventions.[13,14] Only one study of 90 subjects examined a patient-family education intervention.[12] Although only 1 study examined a chronic disease management intervention, this was by far the largest sample size (n = 563).[16]

The use of ESD interventions has continued to receive significant attention.[71] However, there is confusion as to what exactly defines ESD. For example, ESD could be early discharge where the patient gets support after returning home. ESD could also be supported discharge where the support starts early (eg, before discharge) and receives more than just standard care. As we define it for this paper, ESD requires all three components: (1) that the patient is discharged early, (2) that the patient receives support beyond standard of care, and (3) that this support stars before discharge.[11] Before ESD is adopted into practice as an evidence-based approach, these questions need to be addressed.

Despite ESD interventions being the most common across studies, the remaining 4 interventions used in the new studies were carried out on 1063 of the 1690 (63%) participants. In fact the largest sample size focused on a chronic disease management intervention in 563 participants.[16] The 2 community-based support interventions[13,14] (n = 410) included a stroke nurse navigator program that had significant elements of ESD incorporated into the intervention. Likewise, although only the Bodechtel and colleagues[12] study (n = 90) can be discretely categorized as a patient-family educational intervention, several studies (most notably Hohmann and colleagues,[14] Olaiya and colleagues,[16] and Vanacker and colleagues[19]) provide details about education incorporated into the intervention strategy. Despite a repeated call for the need to develop, train, and test transitional care specialists, none of the included interventions could truly be said to provide randomized trial evidence to advance the science of stroke transitional specialists.[72]

Comparator

Although all 9 newly included studies compared an intervention against some form of usual care, there is still no agreed on definition of what constitutes usual care for stroke transitions. As noted by Olson and colleagues,[1] usual care is poorly defined and likely highly variable. Hence, local, regional, national, and global practice diversity creates potential bias and limits external validity when usual care is the default comparator in stroke TOC research. In retrospective trials, the risk of a Hawthorne effect may account for a proportion of the preintervention versus postintervention findings. Although incorporating design elements (eg, block randomization) can reduce this risk, no studies seem to have done so. In prospective trials, there is higher risk of design contamination in which the comparator group is exposed to interventions targeted only for the intervention goup.[73] What is usual is a diverse and complicated set of treatment patterns that are highly dependent on the provider. Although comparing interventions against usual care makes sense for pragmatic designs, there are clear threats to external validity.[74]

Outcome

There is no agreement on what outcome should be targeted as a measure of success in TOC intervention studies. It is difficult to determine if the continued push to develop new and varied outcome measures signals a lack of validity in the current metrics, or simply disparity in agreement as to what functional construct best reflects stroke TOC outcomes. The contribution of validated measures is clearly offset by the heterogeneity of the measures used.[75] The use of individualized outcomes, such as progress toward goal blood pressure, cholesterol, and body mass index, may represent an alternative to a unified measure.[10] Currently the diversity in selecting established outcome measures, and the continued introduction of new measures, significantly limits the generalizability of findings.

Timing

Outcome assessment timing was as diverse as the outcomes assessed (range, 3–12 months). Moreover, we found no association between type of intervention and timing of the outcome assessment. This supports that nurses, who are omnipresent during hospitalization and have high presence and availability in the community, are uniquely positioned to deliver ESD interventions (similar to TOC for cardiovascular patients).[76] The 5 ESD interventions were assessed at 3 different times (2, 3, and 6 months).[15,17–20] The two community-based interventions were assessed at 3 months and 12 months.[13,14] Patient/family education and chronic disease management were assessed at 12 months.[12,16] Unfortunately, this aligns with prior literature on ESD that could not reach consensus on whether interventions should be at fixed intervals (only 60% thought so),[11] and the meaning of "fixed" varies. Likely, unless and until there is agreement on TOC outcome constructs and measures, there will not be agreement on timing of the outcome assessment.

Nursing

Neuroscience nurses have a unique opportunity to contribute to the development of the TOC science and to participate in delivering TOC interventions.[77] Programs have already been developed for several neurologic and neurosurgical conditions in which nurses play leading roles.[78,79] Nurses, by virtue of their bedside presence (in the hospital and in home-care) have a unique lens and training to provide hospital-based and home-based care. Thus, the concept of engaging nurses in transitional-care models is somewhat intuitive.[80]

Limitations

We recognize limitations to this article and the conclusions reached. First, this assessment included only TOC literature for patients with stroke. There is a significant body of literature discussing TOC in general and TOC in nonstroke patients, and the relevance or contribution of this literature to stroke patients is not known. However, a major criticism in the past is that TOC is inherently different based on disease trajectory.[21] This report only included articles discussing stroke TOC from hospital to home, and we do not know how this body of work informs or is informed by stroke TOC between hospital, acute rehabilitation, skilled nursing facility, or other.

Despite 9 new studies, the combined sample includes only 1690 subjects. Moreover, authors noted that they experienced higher than expected loss-to-follow-up and lower than anticipated enrollment rates, and this further limits the generalizability of the results.[12,13,18]

SUMMARY

Little has changed to improve the understanding of best practice for TOC. This evidence summary incorporates findings from 50 studies (41 from the original evidence report and 9 published in the past 8 years). Both patients and their care partners continue to be included as research participants, although the primary focus remains on patients. The focus of TOC research continues to be on interventions falling under the rubric of ESD. The tendency to compare the intervention against a poorly defined usual care group remains ubiquitous. Outcomes constructs can generally be classified as measuring physical functioning, adherence (medication or regimen), and risk reduction (stroke risk factor management). The timing of outcomes remains overly diverse, ranging from 2- to 12-month postdischarge. Future studies should focus on: (1) ESD interventions to improve physical functioning at 12 months, (2) interventions to improve 3- and 12-month medication adherence, (3) sustainable chronic disease management strategies to reduce stroke risk factors at 12 months, and (4) clearly defining care received by the comparator group.

REFERENCES

1. Olson DM, Prvu Bettger J, Alexander KP, et al. Transition of care for acute stroke and myocardial infarction patients: from hospitalization to rehabilitation, recovery, and secondary prevention. Evidence report No. 202. (Prepared by the Duke Evidence-based Practice Center under Contract No. 290-2007-10066-I.) AHRQ Publication No. 11(12)-E011. Rockville (MD): Agency for Healthcare Research and Quality; 2011.
2. Prvu Bettger J, Alexander KP, Dolor RJ, et al. Transitional care after hospitalization for acute stroke or myocardial infarction: a systematic review. Ann Intern Med 2012;157(6):407–16.
3. Benjamin EJ, Blaha MJ, Chiuve SE, et al. Heart disease and stroke statistics-2017 update: a report from the American Heart Association. Circulation 2017;135(10): e146–603.
4. Thrift AG, Thayabaranathan T, Howard G, et al. Global stroke statistics. Int J Stroke 2017;12(1):13–32.
5. Feigin VL, Norrving B, Mensah GA. Global burden of stroke. Circ Res 2017; 120(3):439–48.
6. Jackson N, Haxton E, Morrison K, et al. Reflections on 50 years of neuroscience nursing: the growth of stroke nursing. J Neurosci Nurs 2018;50(4):188–92.
7. Prabhakaran S, Ruff I, Bernstein RA. Acute stroke intervention: a systematic review. JAMA 2015;313(14):1451–62.
8. Mehta N, Watkins D. Stent retrieval devices and time prove beneficial in large vessel occlusions: a synopsis of four recent studies for mechanical retrieval and revascularization. J Neurosci Nurs 2015;47(5):296–9.
9. Ormseth CH, Sheth KN, Saver JL, et al. The American Heart Association's get with the guidelines (GWTG)-Stroke development and impact on stroke care. Stroke Vasc Neurol 2017;2(2):94–105.
10. Agency for Healthcare Research and Quality. Research review title: transition of care for acute stroke and myocardial infarction patients from hospitalization to rehabilitation, recovery, and secondary prevention. Comparative effectiveness research review disposition of comments report 2011. Available at: https://

effectivehealthcare.ahrq.gov/sites/default/files/related_files/stroke-transitions-of-care-disposition-120504.pdf. Accessed December 19, 2018.

11. Fisher RJ, Gaynor C, Kerr M, et al. A consensus on stroke: early supported discharge. Stroke 2011;42(5):1392-7.

12. Bodechtel U, Barlinn K, Helbig U, et al. The stroke east Saxony pilot project for organized post-stroke care: a case-control study. Brain Behav 2016;6(5):e00455.

13. Deen TT T, Kim E, Leahy B, et al. The impact of stroke nurse navigation on patient compliance postdischarge. Rehabil Nurs 2018;43(2):65-72.

14. Hohmann C, Neumann-Haefelin T, Klotz JM, et al. Adherence to hospital discharge medication in patients with ischemic stroke: a prospective, interventional 2-phase study. Stroke 2013;44(2):522-4.

15. Nayeri ND, Mohammadi S, Razi SP, et al. Investigating the effects of a family-centered care program on stroke patients' adherence to their therapeutic regimens. Contemp Nurse 2014;47(1-2):88-96.

16. Olaiya MT, Kim J, Nelson MR, et al. Effectiveness of a shared team approach between nurses and doctors for improved risk factor management in survivors of stroke: a cluster randomized controlled trial. Eur J Neurol 2017;24(7):920-8.

17. Rasmussen RS, Østergaard A, Kjaer P, et al. Stroke rehabilitation at home before and after discharge reduced disability and improved quality of life: a randomised controlled trial. Clin Rehabil 2016;30(3):225-36.

18. Santana S, Rente J, Neves C, et al. Early home-supported discharge for patients with stroke in Portugal: a randomised controlled trial. Clin Rehabil 2017;31(2):197-206.

19. Vanacker P, Standaert D, Libbrecht N, et al. An individualized coaching program for patients with acute ischemic stroke: feasibility study. Clin Neurol Neurosurg 2017;154:89-93.

20. Brown C, Fraser JE, Inness EL, et al. Does participation in standardized aerobic fitness training during inpatient stroke rehabilitation promote engagement in aerobic exercise after discharge? A cohort study. Top Stroke Rehabil 2014;21(Suppl 1):S42-51.

21. Olson DM, Bettger JP, Alexander KP, et al. Transition of care for acute stroke and myocardial infarction patients: from hospitalization to rehabilitation, recovery, and secondary prevention. Evid Rep Technol Assess (Full Rep) 2011;(202):1-197.

22. Bautz-Holter E, Sveen U, Rygh J, et al. Early supported discharge of patients with acute stroke: a randomized controlled trial. Disabil Rehabil 2002;24(7):348-55.

23. Fjaertoft H, Indredavik B, Lydersen S. Stroke unit care combined with early supported discharge: long-term follow-up of a randomized controlled trial. Stroke 2003;34(11):2687-91.

24. Fjaertoft H, Indredavik B, Johnsen R, et al. Acute stroke unit care combined with early supported discharge. Long-term effects on quality of life. A randomized controlled trial. Clin Rehabil 2004;18(5):580-6.

25. Fjaertoft H, Indredavik B, Magnussen J, et al. Early supported discharge for stroke patients improves clinical outcome. Does it also reduce use of health services and costs? One-year follow-up of a randomized controlled trial. Cerebrovasc Dis 2005;19(6):376-83.

26. Indredavik B, Fjaertoft H, Ekeberg G, et al. Benefit of an extended stroke unit service with early supported discharge: a randomized, controlled trial. Stroke 2000;31(12):2989-94.

27. Grasel E, Biehler J, Schmidt R, et al. Intensification of the transition between inpatient neurological rehabilitation and home care of stroke patients. Controlled

clinical trial with follow-up assessment six months after discharge. Clin Rehabil 2005;19(7):725–36.

28. Grasel E, Schmidt R, Biehler J, et al. Long-term effects of the intensification of the transition between inpatient neurological rehabilitation and home care of stroke patients. Clin Rehabil 2006;20(7):577–83.

29. Holmqvist LW, von Koch L, de Pedro-Cuesta J. Use of healthcare, impact on family caregivers and patient satisfaction of rehabilitation at home after stroke in southwest Stockholm. Scand J Rehabil Med 2000;32(4):173–9.

30. von Koch L, Holmqvist LW, Wottrich AW, et al. Rehabilitation at home after stroke: a descriptive study of an individualized intervention. Clin Rehabil 2000;14(6):574–83.

31. von Koch L, de Pedro-Cuesta J, Kostulas V, et al. Randomized controlled trial of rehabilitation at home after stroke: one-year follow-up of patient outcome, resource use and cost. Cerebrovasc Dis 2001;12(2):131–8.

32. Mayo NE, Wood-Dauphinee S, Cote R, et al. There's no place like home: an evaluation of early supported discharge for stroke. Stroke 2000;31(5):1016–23.

33. Teng J, Mayo NE, Latimer E, et al. Costs and caregiver consequences of early supported discharge for stroke patients. Stroke 2003;34(2):528–36.

34. Sulch D, Perez I, Melbourn A, et al. Randomized controlled trial of integrated (managed) care pathway for stroke rehabilitation. Stroke 2000;31(8):1929–34.

35. Sulch D, Evans A, Melbourn A, et al. Does an integrated care pathway improve processes of care in stroke rehabilitation? A randomized controlled trial. Age Ageing 2002;31(3):175–9.

36. Sulch D, Melbourn A, Perez I, et al. Integrated care pathways and quality of life on a stroke rehabilitation unit. Stroke 2002;33(6):1600–4.

37. Torp CR, Vinkler S, Pedersen KD, et al. Model of hospital-supported discharge after stroke. Stroke 2006;37(6):1514–20.

38. Hoffmann T, McKenna K, Worrall L, et al. Randomised trial of a computer-generated tailored written education package for patients following stroke. Age Ageing 2007;36(3):280–6.

39. Clark MS, Rubenach S, Winsor A. A randomized controlled trial of an education and counselling intervention for families after stroke. Clin Rehabil 2003;17(7):703–12.

40. Johnston M, Bonetti D, Joice S, et al. Recovery from disability after stroke as a target for a behavioural intervention: results of a randomized controlled trial. Disabil Rehabil 2007;29(14):1117–27.

41. Mant J, Carter J, Wade DT, et al. Family support for stroke: a randomised controlled trial. Lancet 2000;356(9232):808–13.

42. Mant J, Winner S, Roche J, et al. Family support for stroke: one year follow up of a randomised controlled trial. J Neurol Neurosurg Psychiatry 2005;76(7):1006–8.

43. Sahebalzamani M, Aliloo L, Shakibi A. The efficacy of self-care education on rehabilitation of stroke patients. Saudi Med J 2009;30(4):550–4.

44. Allen KR, Hazelett S, Jarjoura D, et al. Effectiveness of a postdischarge care management model for stroke and transient ischemic attack: a randomized trial. J Stroke Cerebrovasc Dis 2002;11(2):88–98.

45. Allen K, Hazelett S, Jarjoura D, et al. A randomized trial testing the superiority of a postdischarge care management model for stroke survivors. J Stroke Cerebrovasc Dis 2009;18(6):443–52.

46. Wagner EH, Austin BT, Von Korff M. Organizing care for patients with chronic illness. Milbank Q 1996;74(4):511–44.

47. Andersen HE, Schultz-Larsen K, Kreiner S, et al. Can readmission after stroke be prevented? Results of a randomized clinical study: a postdischarge follow-up service for stroke survivors. Stroke 2000;31(5):1038–45.

48. Andersen HE, Eriksen K, Brown A, et al. Follow-up services for stroke survivors after hospital discharge: a randomized control study. Clin Rehabil 2002;16(6): 593–603.

49. Ayana M, Pound P, Lampe F, et al. Improving stroke patients' care: a patient held record is not enough. BMC Health Serv Res 2001;1:1.

50. Boter H. Multicenter randomized controlled trial of an outreach nursing support program for recently discharged stroke patients. Stroke 2004;35(12):2867–72.

51. Claiborne N. Effectiveness of a care coordination model for stroke survivors: a randomized study. Health Soc Work 2006;31(2):87–96.

52. Donnelly M, Power M, Russell M, et al. Randomized controlled trial of an early discharge rehabilitation service: the Belfast Community Stroke Trial. Stroke 2004;35(1):127–33.

53. Ertel KA, Glymour MM, Glass TA, et al. Frailty modifies effectiveness of psychosocial intervention in recovery from stroke. Clin Rehabil 2007;21(6):511–22.

54. Glass TA, Berkman LF, Hiltunen EF, et al. the families in recovery from stroke trial (FIRST): primary study results. Psychosom Med 2004;66(6):889–97.

55. Geddes JM, Chamberlain MA. Home-based rehabilitation for people with stroke: a comparative study of six community services providing co-ordinated, multidisciplinary treatment. Clin Rehabil 2001;15(6):589–99.

56. Mayo NE, Nadeau L, Ahmed S, et al. Bridging the gap: the effectiveness of teaming a stroke coordinator with patient's personal physician on the outcome of stroke. Age Ageing 2008;37(1):32–8.

57. Ricauda NA, Bo M, Molaschi M, et al. Home hospitalization service for acute uncomplicated first ischemic stroke in elderly patients: a randomized trial. J Am Geriatr Soc 2004;52(2):278–83.

58. Torres-Arreola Ldel P, Doubova Dubova SV, Hernandez SF, et al. Effectiveness of two rehabilitation strategies provided by nurses for stroke patients in Mexico. J Clin Nurs 2009;18(21):2993–3002.

59. Joubert J, Reid C, Joubert L, et al. Risk factor management and depression poststroke: the value of an integrated model of care. J Clin Neurosci 2006;13(1): 84–90.

60. Joubert J, Joubert L, Reid C, et al. The positive effect of integrated care on depressive symptoms in stroke survivors. Cerebrovasc Dis 2008;26(2):199–205.

61. Joubert J, Reid C, Barton D, et al. Integrated care improves risk-factor modification after stroke: initial results of the Integrated Care for the Reduction of Secondary Stroke model. J Neurol Neurosurg Psychiatry 2009;80(3):279–84.

62. Askim T, Rohweder G, Lydersen S, et al. Evaluation of an extended stroke unit service with early supported discharge for patients living in a rural community. A randomized controlled trial. Clin Rehabil 2004;18(3):238–48.

63. Askim T, Morkved S, Indredavik B. Does an extended stroke unit service with early supported discharge have any effect on balance or walking speed? J Rehabil Med 2006;38(6):368–74.

64. Cameron JI, O'Connell C, Foley N, et al. Canadian stroke best practice recommendations: managing transitions of care following stroke, guidelines update 2016. Int J Stroke 2016;11(7):807–22.

65. Connolly T, Mahoney E. Stroke survivors' experiences transitioning from hospital to home. J Clin Nurs 2018;27(21–22):3979–87.

66. Kitago T, Ratan RR. Rehabilitation following hemorrhagic stroke: building the case for stroke-subtype specific recovery therapies. F1000Res 2017;6:2044.
67. Alawieh A, Zhao J, Feng W. Factors affecting post-stroke motor recovery: implications on neurotherapy after brain injury. Behav Brain Res 2018;340:94–101.
68. Synhaeve NE, Arntz RM, van Alebeek ME, et al. Women have a poorer very long-term functional outcome after stroke among adults aged 18-50 years: the FUTURE study. J Neurol 2016;263(6):1099–105.
69. Bennett PN, Wang W, Moore M, et al. Care partner: a concept analysis. Nurs Outlook 2017;65(2):184–94.
70. Olson DM. Caregiver or care-partner. J Neurosci Nurs 2017;49(3):136.
71. Cobley CS, Fisher RJ, Chouliara N, et al. A qualitative study exploring patients' and carers' experiences of early supported discharge services after stroke. Clin Rehabil 2013;27(8):750–7.
72. Miller KK, Lin SH, Neville M. From hospital to home to participation: a position paper on transition planning after stroke. Arch Phys Med Rehabil 2018. https://doi.org/10.1016/j.apmr.2018.10.017.
73. Lanspa MJ, Hirshberg EL, Miller RR 3rd, et al. Clinical study replicability and the pursuit of excellence. Crit Care 2015;19:297.
74. Olson DM. What is usual care? J Neurosci Nurs 2019;51(2):61.
75. Maribo T, Nielsen JF, Nielsen CV. Wide variation in function level assessment after stroke in Denmark. Dan Med J 2018;65(10) [pii:A5500].
76. Stoicea N, You T, Eiterman A, et al. Perspectives of post-acute transition of care for cardiac surgery patients. Front Cardiovasc Med 2017;4:70.
77. Magwood GS, White BM, Ellis C. Stroke-related disease comorbidity and secondary stroke prevention practices among young stroke survivors. J Neurosci Nurs 2017;49(5):296–301.
78. Koerner K, Franker L, Douglas B, et al. Disease-specific care: spine surgery program development. J Neurosci Nurs 2017;49(5):286–91.
79. Schneider MA, Schneider MD. Pseudobulbar affect: what nurses, stroke survivors, and caregivers need to know. J Neurosci Nurs 2017;49(2):114–7.
80. Hirschman KB, Shaid E, McCauley K, et al. Continuity of care: the transitional care model. Online J Issues Nurs 2015;20(3):1.

The Projected Transition Trajectory for Survivors and Carers of Patients Who Have Had a Stroke

Norma D. McNair, PhD, RN, ACNS-BC*

KEYWORDS

- Stroke • Transition of care • Carers • Continuity of patient care

KEY POINTS

- Survivors of stroke have a long trajectory of care.
- Poststroke sequelae may include depression, anxiety, and other emotional changes in addition to the physical and cognitive changes that may occur.
- Carers of stroke survivors may have poorer quality of life along with depression and anxiety.
- Research is needed in many areas of poststroke care to identify interventions that may ameliorate the sequelae.

INTRODUCTION

According to the American Heart Association/American Stroke Association, stroke is the fifth leading cause of death in the United States.[1] Every 40 seconds an individual has a stroke and every 4 minutes a person dies as the result of a stroke. Approximately 795,000 individuals suffer a stroke annually in the United States with 610,000 having a new stroke and 185,000 having a recurrent stroke.[2] Globally, there are 10.3 million new strokes annually with higher disability rates in the lower-income and middle-income countries. Disparities between high-income and low-income countries have increased in both the incidence, burden of the costs of care, and disability associated with stroke.[3] The impact of stroke extends beyond the individual who has sustained a stroke. Returning to work may not be possible and the burden to carers and other family members may be substantial.[4]

Disclosure Statement: No conflicts.
Ronald Reagan UCLA Medical Center, Los Angeles, CA, USA
* 2307 Ocean Avenue # 215, Santa Monica, CA 90405.
E-mail address: ndmcnair@twc.com

Nurs Clin N Am 54 (2019) 399–408
https://doi.org/10.1016/j.cnur.2019.04.008
0029-6465/19/© 2019 Elsevier Inc. All rights reserved.

nursing.theclinics.com

ACUTE STROKE CARE

Research has shown that patients cared for in an acute stroke unit have better outcomes than those cared for on nonspecialty units.[4,5] Management of the patient with acute stroke includes ensuring that the guidelines of care are implemented[1] to provide optimal care. These guidelines include a stroke-specific hospital team, early imaging, administration of intravenous alteplase, blood pressure management, temperature, blood glucose, mechanical thrombectomy, and administration of antiplatelets or anticoagulants.[1] Astute nursing care and observation is necessary to ensure that there are no adverse outcomes. **Table 1** outlines the early management of the patient with acute ischemic stroke (AIS).

In 1989, the average length of stay (LOS) for patients with a stroke in an acute setting was approximately 10.2 days. This LOS has decreased to approximately 5.3 days in 2009.[6] This shortened LOS leaves little time for the patient, family, and carers to adjust to the physical and emotional changes that have occurred. Patients and family report that there is a significant adjustment period after a stroke and that information provided in the acute setting is often not recalled.[7,8] Caregivers report an increased burden related to the care of the stroke survivor but also in their own lives as adjustments are made related to care, work, and home lives.[9–12]

Important in the transition from acute care to home is ensuring that information is communicated to all appropriate parties so that care can be seamless. Several transitions of care models have been developed to ensure clear communication of the plan. For example, the Care Transitions Intervention[13] and the Transitional Care[14] models define components that improve transition from the acute care setting to

Table 1	
Guidelines for the care of patients with acute ischemic stroke	
Recommendations	**Interventions**
Early recognition of stroke symptoms	• Call 911 • Education of paramedics and EMS system providers on stroke symptoms
EMS assessment and management	• Field assessment and early intervention by paramedics
Emergency assessment	• Stroke scale assessment • Brain imaging • BP, temperature, and glucose management • IV alteplase • Mechanical thrombectomy • Antiplatelets • Anticoagulants
In-hospital management	• Dedicated stroke unit • BP, temperature, and glucose management • Dysphagia assessment • Nutrition • DVT prophylaxis • Depression screening • Initiate rehabilitation

Abbreviations: BP, blood pressure; DVT, deep vein thrombosis; EMS, emergency medical services; IV, intravenous.

Data from Powers W, Rabinstein A, Ackerson T, et al. 2018 guidelines for the early management of patients with acute ischemic stroke: A guideline for healthcare professionals from the American Heart Association/American Stroke Association. *Stroke.* 2018;49(3).

rehabilitation, skilled nursing facilities, or home. These components include patient and carer engagement, complex medication management, patient and carer education, continuity of care, and accountability from the care team.[14] Coleman and colleagues[13] identified a complete personal health record, transition coach, medication self-management, follow-up, and knowledge of "red flags" as areas of focus. Research has shown that attention to all aspects of transitions of care leads to a decrease in 30-day readmissions and decrease in cost.[15] The Society of Geriatric Medicine[16] in a position statement indicated that care transitions for those with complex medical needs should include preparation of the patient and carer for the next phase of care and communication between all facilities and carers regarding the needs of the patient. In addition, recommendations are made for health care provider education, development of policies that support care transitions, and increased research as to the effectiveness of transition care models.[16]

POST-ACUTE STROKE CARE

Discharge from the acute care setting may lead to placement in rehabilitation, a skilled nursing facility, or home. The goal of care changes from lifesaving to life enhancing. Rehabilitation is designed to assist the survivor in maximizing functional ability and independence. Survivors may spend a few days to several weeks in the rehabilitation setting depending on deficits from the stroke.

The time period for rehabilitation is individual. Some survivors seem to recover quickly and others may take several years. The time frame for recovery depends on the severity of the stroke, type of stroke (acute ischemic vs hemorrhagic), location, and other comorbidities.[17–19] The physical manifestations (hemiplegia/paresis) of the stroke are more readily observed, but some survivors have more difficulty with spatial and cognitive functions, including speech and language, orientation in space, and ability to identify individuals. **Table 2** describes the important interventions in acute rehabilitation. Survivors of stroke face other difficulties that include mood changes and reliance on others to provide care.

Poststroke Depression, Anxiety, and Fatigue

Depression,[20,21] anxiety,[22] and fatigue[23,24] are common after stroke and can inhibit the survivor's ability to fully participate in care. It is often difficult to determine if these issues occur because of the physiologic changes from stroke or because of the physical and emotional manifestations of the stroke.

Poststroke depression

In 1983, the first longitudinal study regarding depression after stroke was published.[25] The results indicated that location of the lesion influenced the severity and frequency of symptoms experienced. The investigators also recognized that depression was multifactorial and included neurophysiological-chemical components in addition to the psychological factors. In several meta-analyses, poststroke depression (PSD) incidence ranged from 39% to 51% within the first 5 years after stroke.[21] Identified risk factors for PSD include age, gender, genetic risk factors, type and severity of stroke, previous psychiatric disorders, location of lesion (left frontal lobe or left basal ganglia), social support, and degree of disability.[21] Cognitive and physical impairment may contribute to PSD.

Of concern in PSD is the risk for higher mortality. In a study published in 1993,[26] 10-year mortality was higher in those with PSD. This was validated in another study.[27] Treatment of PSD with antidepressants has been shown to improve mood and cognitive function in some patients.[28] Other interventions, such as psychotherapy, have

Table 2 Interventions in acute rehabilitation	
Comorbidities	**Interventions**
Prevention of pressure ulcers and contractures	• Risk assessment with valid instrument (eg, Braden scale) • Minimize pressure using approved support surfaces scales • Maintain nutrition, hydration • Daily stretching exercises to affected extremities • Proper positioning of the extremity • Ankle splints at night • Surgical release of contractures may be necessary
DVT prevention	• Prophylactic UFH or LMWH in AIS • Intermittent pneumatic compression • Elastic compression stockings (monitor for skin breakdown)
Bowel and bladder incontinence	• Prompted routine voiding • Pelvic floor exercises • Assessment of bowel function including prestroke routine
Hemiplegic shoulder pain	• Proper positioning of the arm • Shoulder range of motion • Motor retraining • Acupuncture • NMES or TENS • Corticosteroid injection • Botulinum toxin injection • Nerve block • Surgery • Neuromodulating drugs
Central pain	• Pharmacologic interventions • Nonpharmacological interventions
Falls	• Evaluation of risk • Exercise program with ambulation, strength, and balance training • Tai Chi • Home safety evaluation for potential fall risk
Seizures	• Prophylactic AED administration is not recommended • Thorough workup if seizure occurs

Abbreviations: AED, antiepileptic drug; AIS, acute ischemic stroke; DVT, deep vein thrombosis; LMWH, low molecular weight heparin; NMES, neuromuscular electrical stimulation; TENS, transcutaneous electrical stimulation; UHF, unfractionated heparin.

Data from Winstein C, Stein J, Arena R, et al. Guidelines for adult stroke rehabilitation and recovery: A guideline for healthcare professionals from the American Heart Association/American Stroke Association. *Stroke.* 2016;47(6):e98–e169.

been included in studies but have not been shown to be more helpful than a control intervention.[21]

Poststroke anxiety

Anxiety is a common mental health condition in the United States,[29] and its prevalence after stroke is approximately 20% to 25%. Anxiety is more common in women, younger stroke survivors, those from lower-income backgrounds, and those unable to return to work after the stroke.[29] Interventions for poststroke anxiety (PSA) are not well studied. Guidelines are available for treating anxiety in the general population but these do not focus on PSA. Recommendations for treatment of PSA include medication (serotonin reuptake inhibitors, tricyclic antidepressants, benzodiazepines, and hypnotics), psychological therapy (behavior therapy, cognitive therapy, or cognitive-behavioral therapy) and complementary or alternative therapies (yoga, other exercise, relaxation therapy).[29] There are no randomized controlled trials examining any of these treatments, dosage, or their effectiveness in survivors of stroke.

Poststroke fatigue

Poststroke fatigue (PSF) is common after stroke, with as many as half of stroke survivors experiencing it. Some estimates of PSF are as high as 75%. Definitions of fatigue are general and are not specific to those who have survived a stroke. It has been suggested that PSF is multifactorial and includes the following: medication, smoking, physical and medical comorbidities, demographics, prestroke fatigue, sleep disturbances, depression, and anxiety.[23] It has been theorized that PSF occurs as a result of inflammation, immune response, and genetic makeup, but research that has been completed has included small sample sizes and nonrandomized samples. Research in the field of biomarkers that might identify PSF is still in its infancy.[23,30] It is unclear if PSF is a result of injury to the brain at the time of the stroke or some other mechanism. Because fatigue is also present in depression, it is important to differentiate the cause of fatigue and direct treatment accordingly. Research into PSF is sparse and is needed to identify causes and treatment.

Long-Term Outcomes After Stroke

Few studies have examined long-term outcomes after stroke; however, research has been conducted on health-related quality of life (HRQoL) after stroke. One study, conducted 6 months poststroke, indicated that quality of life (QOL) was lower than in those in the general population, and that age, being female, presence of social support, previous history of stroke, and disabilities influenced QOL.[31]

Another study examined HRQoL within the first 6 months after a stroke and unmet needs at 2 years poststroke.[32] Results indicated that reduced HRQoL in the early months after stroke lead to more unmet needs at 2 years. These needs included community reintegration and meaningful roles in the context of the disability. Additional unmet needs were in the physical and emotional arenas. These unmet needs were categorized as being able to participate in activities, mobility, self-care, pain, anxiety, and depression.[32] These investigators suggested that more research is needed to identify HRQoL early after stroke and possible interventions that would decrease unmet needs long-term.

Researchers in Japan examined home-dwelling stroke survivors 1 to 3 years after stroke. Results indicated that activities of daily living (ADLs) and depression affected HRQoL. The investigators recommended that emphasis be placed on ADLs early in the inpatient rehabilitation phase to improve long-term HRQoL.[20]

De Wit and colleagues,[33] in a multicenter European study, examined the impact of stroke on survivors 5 years after stroke. Results indicated that HRQoL was lower 5 years poststroke than that of the general population. In addition, survivors with higher levels of depression, anxiety, and disability were associated with lower HRQoL. The investigators recommended that survivors have longer-term follow-up post inpatient rehabilitation to attempt to ameliorate some of these sequelae of stroke.

Longitudinal studies exist, but few follow stroke survivors for longer than 24 months. Recommendations from these longer-term studies include the need to continue rehabilitation long after the inpatient rehabilitation phase is completed.[17,34] One study found that 70% of stroke survivors were disabled or had died at 5 years poststroke. The investigators indicated that more improvements are needed in immediate poststroke care and in secondary stroke prevention to improve these outcomes[34] (**Table 3**).

Table 3
Secondary stroke prevention

Risk Factors	Interventions
Hypertension	• BP therapy in previously untreated survivors • Maintain BP at systolic ≤140 mm Hg and diastolic ≤90 mm Hg • Resumption of BP therapy in previously treated survivors • Lifestyle changes
Dyslipidemia	• Statin therapy • Treat according to guidelines
Glucose and diabetes management	• Screen for diabetes • Treat according to guidelines
Overweight/Obesity	• Measure BMI
Metabolic syndrome	• For those with metabolic syndrome, lifestyle modification should be addressed
Physical inactivity	• For those who are able, moderate to vigorous exercise 3–4 times/wk • Those with disability should be supervised by a professional at the initiation of a program
Nutrition	• Nutritional assessment • Mediterranean-type diet • Sodium reduction to ≤2.4 g/d
Obstructive sleep apnea	• Sleep study • Treatment with CPAP
Tobacco use	• Advise survivors to quit • Provide resources for support • Avoid passive smoke
Alcohol use	• Heavy users should decrease use • Moderate users (2 drinks/day) may be reasonable to continue • Nonusers should not start drinking
Atrial fibrillation	• Long-term cardiac monitoring may be useful in detecting atrial fibrillation • VKA therapy (apixaban, dabigatran); target INR 2.5 • Prevention of recurrence (rivaroxaban) • For patients with known CAD, anticoagulation and antiplatelet therapy may be beneficial • For those unable to tolerate oral anticoagulants, aspirin or aspirin + clopidogrel may be helpful

Abbreviations: BMI, body mass index; BP, blood pressure; CAD, coronary artery disease; CPAP, continuous positive airway pressure; INR, international normalized ratio; VKA, vitamin K antagonist.

Data from Jönsson A-C, Höglund P, Brizzi M, Pessah-Rasmussen H. Secondary prevention and health promotion after stroke: can it be enhanced? J Stroke Cerebrovasc Dis. 2014;23(9):2287–2295.

CARER SUPPORT

Survivors of stroke often require care after discharge from acute rehabilitation. Informal carers, in the form of family members, are often enlisted. Often, these family members do not have the skills and knowledge to provide daily care and their needs are usually not addressed in the poststroke acute period. Research has shown that carer burden can lead to depression, anxiety, and a change in QOL in both the survivor and the carer.[12,35–37]

Longitudinal studies have indicated that burden and QOL vary over time. The time for highest burden seems to be in the first 3 to 6 months poststroke, with improvement at 12 months or more. Carer QOL seems to be related to the physical functioning of the survivor. If the survivor is more disabled, the carer experiences more burden, including depression and anxiety.[12] The investigators of this study recommend ensuring that both the survivor and the carer are educated together in preparation for caregiving.

A study using an online and telephone intervention, in a population of veterans, examined the length of time of caregiving and burden experienced. The time of caregiving ranged from 2 months to 46.5 years. The results indicated that burden and depression were negatively related to the length of time of caregiving. In addition, interventions directed at relieving burden and depression led to an improvement in symptoms.[35]

Carer burden has been identified in many situations in which informal carers assist a family member.[38–40] Information from these studies may identify interventions that would be applicable to the survivor of stroke and their carer.

RESEARCH IMPLICATIONS

Research, especially research conducted by nurses, is needed in stroke. Several areas need more robust, randomized controlled trials. Outlined as follows are potential research topics for the nurse interested in the care of survivors of stroke and their carers.

Acute stroke care
- Effectiveness of stroke units on outcomes[31]
- Effectiveness of stroke guidelines on LOS and outcomes[1]
- Patient and carer retention of education related to discharge[19]
- Use of teach-back and health literacy assessment for survivors and carers[7,8]
- Transitions of care models that are effective for survivors of stroke, including important elements[15,16]

Post-acute stroke care
- Effectiveness of rehabilitation guidelines in care improvement[41]

Poststroke Depression, Anxiety, and Fatigue
- Causes of poststroke depression, anxiety, and fatigue[26,29,30]
- Differentiation of these from that of the general population[29,30]
- Effectiveness of interventions to treat depression, anxiety, and fatigue[26–30]

Long-term outcomes
- HRQoL in survivors of stroke and carers[20,32]
- Longitudinal studies beyond 2 years after stroke[34]
- Effectiveness of secondary stroke prevention and lifestyle changes for survivors and carers[33]
- Interventions that might relieve carer burden and enhance QOL[34]

Carer burden care
- Support needed for carers[38–40]
- Longer-term follow-up with carers to examine QOL and burden, depression, and anxiety[38–40]

CLINICAL IMPLICATIONS FOR NURSING

Nurses provide treatment to patients with stroke over a continuum of care, beginning in the prehospital phase, through the emergency department, acute care, and rehabilitation. Often, after the survivor is discharged from rehabilitation, follow-up occurs in the home with home health services and in the provider's clinic for medical care. Little research has been conducted on the role of the nurse in the post-acute care settings.

One study advocated for a nurse practitioner in the clinic to reduce 30-day readmissions after a stroke. In this study, readmission rates were decreased by 48% with a combination of early posthospital clinic appointments and discharge phone calls.[41] Rehabilitation nurses have been identified as having a significant contribution to ensuring that stroke survivors and their families and carers are ready for discharge. Camicia and colleagues[42] document the essential role of the rehabilitation nurse and recommends for nurses to be involved in policy and research to advocate for the patient. Unfortunately, research in the role of the nurse in home health management in stroke is limited.

In summary, survivors of stroke embark on a life-long journey of recovery and navigate many emotions and physical limitations in an effort to have a good QOL. Carers also need assistance and education that will allow them to have a good QOL. Nurses can assist in the transition from acute care to home and ensure that families and survivors are prepared for each transition. More research is necessary to evaluate the role of the nurse in all of these settings. In addition, research is needed to determine the needs of family members, carers, and the stroke survivor for the long-term.

REFERENCES

1. Powers W, Rabinstein A, Ackerson T, et al. 2018 guidelines for the early management of patients with acute ischemic stroke: a guideline for healthcare professionals from the American Heart Association/American Stroke Association. Stroke 2018;49(3):e46–110.
2. Benjamin EJ, Virani SS, Callaway CW, et al. Heart disease and stroke statistics 2018 update: a report from the American Heart Association. Circulation 2018; 137(12):e67–492.
3. Pandian J, Gall S, Kate M, et al. Prevention of stroke: a global perspective. Lancet 2018;392(10154):1269–78.
4. Wissel J, Olver J, Sunnerhagen K. Navigating the poststroke continuum of care. J Stroke Cerebrovasc Dis 2013;22(1):1–8.
5. Stroke Unit Trialists' Collaboration. Organised inpatient (stroke unit) care for stroke. Cochrane Database Syst Rev 2013;(9):CD000197.
6. Hall M, Levant S, DeFrances C. Hospitalization for stroke in U.S. hospitals, 1989–2009. NCHS Data Brief 2012;95:1–8.
7. Cameron V. Best practices for stroke patient and family education in the acute care setting: a literature review. Medsurg Nurs 2013;22(1):51–5.
8. Roy D, Gasquoine S, Caldwell S, et al. Health professional and family perceptions of post-stroke information. Nurs Prax N Z 2015;31(2):7–24.
9. Carod-Artal F, Egido J. Quality of life after stroke: the importance of a good recovery. Cerebrovasc Dis 2009;27(Suppl 1):204–14.
10. Kruithof W, Post M, van Mierlo M, et al. Caregiver burden and emotional problems in partners of stroke patients at two months and one year post-stroke: determinants and prediction. Patient Educ Couns 2016;99(10):1632–40.
11. Pont W, Groeneveld I, Arwert H, et al. Caregiver burden after stroke: changes over time? Disabil Rehabil 2018. [Epub ahead of print].
12. Pucciarelli G, Vellone E, Savini S, et al. Roles of changing physical function and caregiver burden on quality of life in stroke: a longitudinal dyadic analysis. Stroke 2017;48(3):733–9.

13. Coleman E, Smith J, Frank J, et al. Preparing patients and caregivers to partici-
    pate in care delivered across settings: The Care Transitions Intervention. J Am
    Geriatr Soc 2004;52(11):1817–25.
14. Naylor M, Shaid E, Carpenter D, et al. Components of comprehensive and effec-
    tive transitional care. J Am Geriatr Soc 2017;65(6):1119–25.
15. Davidson G, Austin E, Thornblade L, et al. Improving transitions of care across
    the spectrum of healthcare delivery: a multidisciplinary approach to understand-
    ing variability in outcomes across hospitals and skilled nursing facilities. Am J
    Surg 2017;213(5):910–4.
16. Coleman E, Boult C. Improving the quality of transitional care for persons with
    complex care needs: position statement of The American Geriatrics Society
    Health Care Systems Committee. J Am Geriatr Soc 2003;51(4):556–7.
17. Arntzen C, Borg T, Hamran T. Long-term recovery trajectory after stroke: an
    ongoing negotiation between body, participation and self. Disabil Rehabil 2015;
    37(18):1626–34.
18. Chan L, Sandel M, Jette A, et al. Does postacute care site matter? A longitudinal
    study assessing functional recovery after a stroke. Arch Phys Med Rehabil 2013;
    94(4):622–9.
19. Connolly T, Mahoney E. Stroke survivors' experiences transitioning from hospital
    to home. J Clin Nurs 2018;27(21–22):3979–87.
20. Mutai H, Furukawa T, Nakanishi K, et al. Longitudinal functional changes, depres-
    sion, and health-related quality of life among stroke survivors living at home after
    inpatient rehabilitation. Psychogeriatrics 2016;16(3):185–90.
21. Robinson R, Jorge R. Post-stroke depression: a review. Am J Psychiatry 2016;
    173(3):221–31.
22. Maaijwee N, Tendolkar I, Rutten-Jacobs L, et al. Long-term depressive symptoms
    and anxiety after transient ischaemic attack or ischaemic stroke in young adults.
    Eur J Neurol 2016;23(8):1262–8.
23. Hinkle J, Becker K, Kim J, et al. Poststroke fatigue: emerging evidence and ap-
    proaches to management: a scientific statement for healthcare professionals
    from the American Heart Association. Stroke 2017;48(7):e159–70.
24. Wu S, Kutlubaev M, Chun H, et al. Interventions for post-stroke fatigue. Cochrane
    Database Syst Rev 2015;7.
25. Robinson R, Starr L, Kubos K, et al. A two-year longitudinal study of post-stroke
    mood disorders: findings during the initial evaluation. Stroke 1983;14(5):736–41.
26. Morris PL, Robinson RG, Andrzejewski P, et al. Association of depression with 10-
    year poststroke mortality. Am J Psychiatry 1993;150(1):124–9.
27. House A, Knapp P, Bamford J, et al. Mortality at 12 and 24 months after stroke
    may be associated with depressive symptoms at 1 month. Stroke 2001;32(3):
    696–701.
28. Kimura M, Robinson R, Kosier J. Treatment of cognitive impairment after post-
    stroke depression: a double-blind treatment trial. Stroke 2000;31(7):1482–6.
29. Knapp P, Campbell Burton C, Holmes J, et al. Interventions for treating anxiety
    after stroke. Cochrane Database Syst Rev 2017;(5):CD008860.
30. De Doncker W, Dantzer R, Ormstad H, et al. Mechanisms of poststroke fatigue.
    J Neurol Neurosurg Psychiatry 2018;89:287–93.
31. Lopez-Espuela F, Pedrera Zamorano J, Ramırez-Moreno J, et al. Determinants of
    quality of life in stroke survivors after 6 months, from a comprehensive stroke unit:
    a longitudinal study. Biol Res Nurs 2015;17(5):461–8.

32. Andrew N, Kilkenny M, Lannin N, et al. Is health-related quality of life between 90 and 180 days following stroke associated with long-term unmet needs? Qual Life Res 2016;25:2053–62.
33. De Wit L, Theuns P, Dejaeger E, et al. Long-term impact of stroke on patients' health-related quality of life. Disabil Rehabil 2017;39(14):1435–40.
34. Luengo-Fernandez R, Paul N, Gray A, et al. Population-based study of disability and institutionalization after transient ischemic attack and stroke: 10-year results of the Oxford Vascular Study. Stroke 2013;44:2854–61.
35. Graf R, LeLaurin J, Schmitzberger M, et al. The stroke caregiving trajectory in relation to caregiver depressive symptoms, burden, and intervention outcomes. Top Stroke Rehabil 2017;24(7):488–95.
36. Pucciarelli G, Ausili D, Galbussera A, et al. Quality of life, anxiety, depression and burden among stroke caregivers: a longitudinal, observational multicentre study. J Adv Nurs 2018;74(8):1875–87.
37. Pucciarelli G, Lee C, Lyons K, et al. Quality of life trajectories among stroke survivors and the related changes in caregiver outcomes: a growth mixture study. Arch Phys Med Rehabil 2019;100(3):433–40.e1.
38. Al-Daken L, Ahmad M. Predictors of burden and quality of sleep among family caregivers of patients with cancer. Support Care Cancer 2018;26(11):3967–73.
39. Kajiwara K, Noto H, Yamanaka M. Changes in caregiving appraisal among family caregivers of persons with dementia: a longitudinal study over 12 months. Psychogeriatrics 2018;18(6):460–7.
40. Mosley P, Moodie R, Dissanayaka N. Caregiver burden in Parkinson disease: a critical review of recent literature. J Geriatr Psychiatry Neurol 2017;30(5):235–52.
41. Condon C, Lycan S, Duncan P, et al. Reducing readmissions after stroke with a structured nurse practitioner/registered nurse transitional stroke program. Stroke 2016;47(6):1599–604.
42. Camicia M, Black T, Farrell J, et al. The essential role of the rehabilitation nurse in facilitating care transitions: a white paper by the Association of Rehabilitation Nurses. Rehabil Nurs 2014;39(1):3–15.

The Transition Trajectory for the Patient with a Traumatic Brain Injury

Ava M. Puccio, RN, PhD[a],*, Maighdlin W. Anderson, DNP, ACNP-BC[b],
Anita Fetzick, RN, MSN, CCNS[a]

KEYWORDS

• Traumatic brain injury • Acute care • Discharge status • Complications • Outcome

KEY POINTS

- The trajectory of patients with traumatic brain injury is discussed.
- Acute hospitalization and discharge status of these patients is explained.
- Medications for and complications of traumatic brain injury are discussed.
- Functional and neurologic outcomes are delineated.

INITIAL EMERGENCY ROOM VISIT AND HOSPITALIZATION

The acute and subacute trajectories of the patient with a traumatic brain injury (TBI) varies by the initial triage of the brain injury, with the description of the injury (type, velocity), initial symptoms, and level of consciousness dictating the course of acute care decision making. Approximately 1.7 million people suffer a TBI each year, with an estimated 1.5 million deaths and more than 55 million people living with the sequelae of TBI to some degree.[1] The American Congress of Rehabilitation Medicine criteria for a head computed tomography (CT) scan after a head injury is followed by the majority of trauma centers, resulting in a low predicted threshold for a CT scan to be performed.[2] The results of this scan then informs hospital bed assignment. A negative CT scan for neurologic injury, and no other injuries or symptoms will most likely result in an emergency department (ED) discharge. A positive CT scan will most likely warrant at least a 1-night stay with a repeat head CT to ensure no expansion of the CT abnormality. Apart from the CT scan results, the level of consciousness (Glasgow

Disclosure Statement: Dr A.M. Puccio receives support from NIH/NINR R00 NR013176. Other authors have nothing to disclose.
[a] Department of Neurological Surgery, Neurotrauma Clinical Trials Center, University of Pittsburgh, 200 Lothrop Street, Suite B-400, Pittsburgh, PA 15213, USA; [b] University of Pittsburgh School of Nursing, 324 Victoria Building, 3500 Victoria Street, Pittsburgh, PA 15261, USA
* Corresponding author.
E-mail address: puccioam@upmc.edu

Coma Scale [GCS]) and physical examination dictates the level of nursing care that is needed and ultimately determines admission to the intensive care unit (ICU).

Concern for follow-up of the with a TBI is seen for all severities of injury. Patients discharged from the ED are often instructed that a few days of rest is all that is needed for recovery and may or may not be provided instruction if postconcussive symptoms arise or are not resolved. In these cases, it is up to the patient and their family to decide if symptoms are normal and when to seek additional medical care. It has been shown with a large cohort of patients with a TBI from 3 high-acuity level 1 institutions enrolling in the Transforming Research and Clinical Knowledge in Traumatic Brain Injury (TRACK-TBI) study that approximately 33% of patients with a mild TBI at 3 months after the injury were functionally impaired (Glasgow Outcome Scale-Extended score of ≤6) and 22.4% remained below full functional status at 1 year.[3] These percentages have been validated in larger cohorts and special populations; in addition, females have been shown to have 3 times the percentage of depressive symptoms and lack of return to work.[4] Discharge instructions should provide frequently asked questions (and their answers) about postconcussive care and follow-up information. For patients who are admitted to the hospital, trauma services may direct follow-up care and may or may not include concussive follow-up information. Once again, this TBI population should be provided frequently asked questions and answers about postconcussive care as well as follow-up information. Activity restrictions should be discussed and instructed depending on the severity of injury, and preinjury status. For teens, discharge plans should include return to play (sports injuries) and return to school (potential altered classes). The discharge plans for an adult with a TBI should discuss return to work, driving, and exercise. The elderly patient has additional concerns, because they may not have been followed recently by a primary care physician and their prehospital status may have a large influence on the follow-up care; many activities of daily living may be affected. A formal driving evaluation should be recommended.[5] Unique aspects of a rural home environment, with terrain concerns, limited transportation accessibility, limited communication, and a lack of TBI education of health care providers should also be considered.

Evaluation of the Patient with a Severe Traumatic Brain Injury (Prehospital and Emergency Department)

Prehospital management using the American College of Surgeons Advanced Trauma Life Support guidelines[6] is critical during the initial resuscitation and treatment of trauma patients. Spine stabilization during transport with a neck collar and backboard is critical to prevent spinal cord injury and also promotes correct neck alignment for optimal cerebral perfusion pressure and venous return. In addition, specific to the head injury population, the use of short-acting neuromuscular paralytic agents for intubation of the patient allows a fast triage and assessment of neurologic impairment (an accurate GCS score) upon hospital arrival. The management of the suspected head injured patient should include the conservative use of hyperventilation (to promote cerebral blood flow) and avoidance of mannitol (to avoid volume-depleting diuretic effect), and steroids. Efficient and quick trauma assessments allow for neurosurgical candidates to be treated immediately. Approximately 25% of patients with a severe TBI admitted to a level 1 institution require an emergent craniotomy for evacuation of intracranial mass lesions (hematomas, large contusions). This emergent nature of treatment justifies the transfer of a patient with a severe TBI to a level 1 triage hospital for the advanced care, which is staffed by trained nursing and medical personnel, in particular, in-house neurosurgeons and a dedicated trauma operating room.

After stabilization in the ED and confirmation of severity of injury by an attending neurosurgeon or, in an academic setting, a trained neurotrauma resident in consultation with the attending neurosurgeon, a patient with severe a TBI is transferred to a dedicated neurotrauma ICU. Initial examination of the injured patient, either at the scene of the accident, or upon admission to the hospital cannot accurately predict long-term outcome, providing reason to treat all patients aggressively. The primary goal of caring for the trauma patient with a head injury is the prevention of secondary brain injury, a major determinant in overall neurologic outcome. Prehospital, emergency room, and acute care treatment, as well as rehabilitative services are coordinated to reflect current *Guidelines for the Management of Severe Head Injuries*, produced by the Brain Trauma Foundation.[7]

An interdisciplinary approach is immediately instituted once the patient arrives in the ED with coordinated care with neurosurgery, trauma services, and critical care medicine, as well as early involvement of physical and occupational therapy and rehabilitative services. Standardized clinical orders with adherence to the *Guidelines for the Treatment of Severe Traumatic Brain injury* published by the Brain Trauma Foundation are implemented to minimize individualized physician ideologies.[7] All standing orders are focused on the minimization or prevention of secondary injury occurring within this acute recovery period, with an emphasis of oxygenation and blood flow. This consistency in standing orders and implementation by dedicated brain trauma nurses ensures that all patients with a severe TBI are treated equally aggressive. The trajectory of care in the ICU will be heavily dependent on the severity of the brain injury (as assessed with GCS and neurologic examination) as well as any confounding factors such as other traumatic injuries, preexisting conditions, advanced age, or intoxication with drugs or alcohol. Additional injuries and disease processes will all increase the risk of complications and the length of ICU stay. Ventilatory support is given through an endotracheal tube or a tracheostomy for patients who are unable to protect their airway, either from low levels of consciousness or traumatic injuries. With ventilatory support, especially if extended, comes an increased risk of pneumonia as well as other pulmonary problems and complications. The risk of ventilator-associated pneumonia within the first 14 days of intubation is estimated at 1.5% each day and is the leading cause of death from nosocomial infections in critically ill patients.[8,9] The prevalence of acute respiratory distress syndrome is common after a severe TBI with rates of 30% and higher. Patients with acute respiratory distress syndrome have significantly longer lengths of ICU and hospital stays.[10]

Acute care monitoring for patients with a severe TBI is extensive. Intracranial monitoring is warranted for all patients with a severe TBI defined as a GCS score of 8 or less, not following commands, without the influence of paralytics and sedation. Intracranial pressure (ICP) monitoring should be measured regularly, either continuously or hourly through either an extraventricular drain or an intraparenchymal catheter.[7] The goal is to control ICP to less than or equal to 22 mm Hg with treatment in a stepwise escalation of therapy, with head position, sedation, analgesia, and mannitol and/or hypertonic saline.[7] If there is no response with these therapies, persistent intracranial hypertension can be treated with the addition of neuromuscular blockade and moderate hyperventilation (to a P_{CO_2} of 29–31 mm Hg). In the cases of refractory ICP, early decisions for decompressive craniectomy can be made. If a patient is not a surgical candidate, or if refractory ICP occurs after a decompressive craniectomy, a pentobarbital coma is a consideration. Additional monitoring for patients with a severe TBI is brain tissue oxygen and temperature monitoring and local blood flow probes. This monitoring is placed via a bolt catheter.

The length of ICP monitoring is variable, with peak ICP elevations within 72 hours after a severe TBI.[11] After the removal of the ICP monitoring, a follow-up CT scan should be performed before hospital discharge to evaluate posttraumatic hydrocephalus, a known complication in approximately 11% of all patients with a severe TBI, and a higher incidence risk of 6 times or greater in those patients requiring a decompressive craniectomy.[12]

Hospital Discharge and Follow-Up

Discharge disposition

Recovery after a brain injury, especially a severe TBI, is a long process. Owing to this span across time, the coordination of care is important for optimal neurologic recovery. With the advancement of medical interventions in the early phase of TBI, there has been an improvement in the survival rate, with an increased number of patients requiring long-term management of disabilities resulting from an injury.[13,14] Nurses should be educated on the predictors of discharge disposition early in the recovery period so that a realistic plan of care can be developed within a timely fashion. A rehabilitation specialist should be consulted early in the acute hospitalization and incorporated in the daily rounds and care of patients with a severe TBI. This process of rehabilitation starts early in the ICU or hospital ward, where issues such as swallowing, spasticity, mobility, and neurobehavioral disorders are evaluated by clinicians, and may prompt interdisciplinary consultation with physiatry.

Families and caregivers should be involved in assessment of postacute needs. The process also allows for the rehabilitation specialist to assess the course of recovery and the potential for the patient to participate in rehabilitation therapies upon discharge from the acute care setting. It is important to conservatively use days within a rehabilitation facility allotted by insurance companies. Although most patients with TBI are discharged to home, patients with a severe TBI are likely to be discharged initially to a skilled nursing facility for postacute care based on their neurologic status (e.g., not following commands). In addition, a patient with a TBI may not be able to participate in rehabilitative therapies if the patient also has polytrauma that does not allow weight-bearing status. Follow-up with a neurotrauma specialist within the first 6 months after discharge assists in ensuring proper referrals are performed and coordinated. For instance, if complications or improvements occur in the skilled nursing facility or rehabilitation setting, the patients may need to be readmitted to an acute hospital (i.e., shunt evaluation, repeat head CT scan). Although families may strive for a discharge to home, special adaptations after a severe TBI, even with the best outcomes, are often required. Vocational rehabilitation assists in a successful transition to a better quality of living at home after hospitalization for a TBI.[15] There are several possibilities for discharge disposition in TBI, and selection of the appropriate setting requires a multidisciplinary approach (**Table 1**).[16]

Discharge medication management At discharge from the hospital, many patients will have medication plans that are markedly different than their prehospital regimens. As with patients with other diagnoses, chronic conditions such as diabetes and hypertension can be newly diagnosed in patients with a TBI and they will need education specific to those problems. Unlike the majority of other patients, however, most patients with a moderate or severe TBI will also need specific and tailored education about anticoagulation medications and antiseizure medications, if prescribed (either prophylactic or for treatment) by the trauma/neurosurgery team upon discharge and follow-up.

Table 1
Discharge settings and predictors

Discharge Setting	Predictors of Discharge[16]
Home	Most patients with TBI are discharged to home • Patients generally desire discharge to home • Patients may lack the support to access rehabilitation or skilled services based on insurance coverage
Inpatient rehabilitation	Younger adults are more likely to be discharged to inpatient rehabilitation Patients with higher injury severity or increased length of stay are more likely to be discharged to rehabilitation facilities
Skilled nursing facility or long-term acute care facility	Older adults are more likely to be discharged to skilled nursing facilities • May be eligible for Medicare insurance to allow for coverage of services • Older patients have relatively higher medical frailty and more comorbidities

From Zarshenas S, Tam L, Colantonio A, Alavinia SM, Cullen N. Predictors of discharge destination from acute care in patients with traumatic brain injury. *BMJ open.* 2017;7(8):e016694.

Anticoagulation and antiplatelet therapy   Anticoagulants and antiplatelets are used to prevent and treat thromboembolism as well as to prevent the formation of clots on vessel walls and along artificial valves. In patients with atrial fibrillation, these medications can greatly decrease the risk of stroke; for patients with a physiologic tendency to form clots, they can prevent pulmonary embolisms and deep vein thromboses. In the setting of a TBI, however, anticoagulation increases overall mortality,[17] and the replacement of blood clotting factors as well as the reversal of medication is of utmost importance early in the course of the injury. Once all components of the injury start to stabilize, including areas of contusion, ischemia, or intracranial hemorrhage, the decision about when to restart anticoagulation or antiplatelet therapy must be made. There are no national guidelines or consensus about the optimal timing for restarting anticoagulation but, in general, in able patients who are not at high risk for repeated falls or trauma, there is a net benefit in terms of reduction of risk of thromboembolic events despite the increased risk of intracranial hemorrhage.[18] Many clinicians will restart anticoagulation in the ICU, first using an easily reversible heparin in intravenous infusion form while they continue high-intensity neurologic monitoring. If the patient remains neurologically stable, the transition to long-acting oral anticoagulants proceeds before leaving the hospital. For certain high-risk conditions, such as artificial valves, aspirin may be started as soon as the patient is stable, before leaving the hospital. In the absence of an extremely high risk for thrombus formation, however, antiplatelet medications may be held for several weeks to months to allow time for greater stabilization of intracranial vessels and healing of fragile areas of injury.

Once out of the hospital, whether at home or in a rehabilitation or nursing center, extra precautions to avoid falls need to be taken to avoid causing any new intracranial bleeding. Close monitoring of laboratory tests and medication dosages is usually done by a primary care physician or cardiologist. The neurosurgery team may schedule more frequent follow-up appointments in the beginning of the postacute phase owing to the higher risk for dangerous intracranial bleeding associated with anticoagulation after a TBI.

Antiseizure medications   Posttraumatic seizures (PTS) are a known complication of TBI.[19] They can be categorized as early (within 7 days of injury) or late (occurring after the first 7 days after the injury). Common management for many years was to treat with phenytoin prophylactically from the time of admission to the hospital for a week to many months, depending on clinical judgment, to prevent early and late PTS. Multiple studies, however, showed that seizure prophylaxis with phenytoin reduced early PTS in patients with a severe TBI, but did not affect the probability of late PTS or improve overall outcomes.[20,21] Later studies showed equivalent outcomes for levetiracetam, making it another choice for seizure prophylaxis for patients with a severe TBI.[22,23] The Guidelines for the Management of Severe TBI, 4th edition, have a Level IIa recommendation to use phenytoin for 7 days to decrease risk of early PTS only and do not see sufficient evidence to recommend levetiracetam over phenytoin.[7]

In the setting of seizure activity during that 7 days, antiepileptic medications would be titrated to stop seizure activity and continued under the supervision of a neurologist as an outpatient. Patients with recorded or observed seizures would ideally be transitioned to a medium- to long-acting oral antiepileptic such as levetiracetam upon discharge from the hospital.

Pain, anxiety, and sleep medications   Early in the treatment course after severe or moderate TBI, patients may receive opioid analgesics, either as a part of a sedation package (along with propofol) to treat intracranial hypertension or to treat pain related to their traumatic injuries and head injuries, as well as other types of traumatic injuries or postsurgical pain. Ideally, this medication is decreased and eventually weaned off as soon as possible and the goal is to be off all opioid pain medications before discharge from the hospital. In an isolated TBI (no other traumatic injuries) this goal is reachable, but there are often situations, especially in polytrauma, where patients are discharged with an opioid prescription to treat the remnants of acute pain while they rehabilitate.[24] The goal in this case would be to prescribe the lowest possible dose that also relieves pain and to coordinate follow-up with a pain specialist or their primary care doctor to ensure that alternative methods for pain control are recommended and that opioid medications are discontinued appropriately when pain is more controlled with other adjuvant therapies.[24]

Anxiolytics and sleep aids are not often started in the hospital for patients with a TBI and the problems of anxiety and insomnia are not usually seen during the acute course of a TBI. Both insomnia and anxiety, however, can be problems for people recovering from severe and moderate, as well as mild, TBI. Methods for self-treatment and self-management may be learned during rehabilitation or later as the problems begin to arise. Discharge planning for and coordination of strategies for treatment are often lacking and further nursing research is needed.

Neurologic outcome and functional evaluations   After a TBI, both functional and neurologic status is assessed at follow-up clinic appointments depending on the initial injury severity and outcome. In cases of mild TBI, symptomology is often assessed via questionnaire or computer-based assessment tools. The Brief Symptom Inventory-18[25] assesses psychological distress by obtaining self-report on somatization and depression and anxiety symptoms. Each dimension contains 6 questions. They are evaluated via rating the level of distress over the past 7 days in each category from 0 to 4 on Likert-type scale, with 4 being extremely often. In tests of validity, the Brief Symptom Inventory correlates significantly with other validated psychosocial and functional tests in patients with a TBI.[26] The Immediate Post-Concussion and Cognitive Testing test[27] is an example of a computer-based neurocognitive assessment tool that is commonly implemented in concussion clinics and for sports trainers assessments. It consists of 15- to 20-minute assessments of psychomotor function, processing speed, attention, learning, memory, and working memory that are based on keystroke responses to visual stimuli presented on a computer screen and has been shown to have reliability and sensitivity. Functional outcome after a TBI is often assessed and scored using the Glasgow Outcome Scale,[28] a global measure assessing the level of disability after acute brain injury by using broad categories: good recovery, moderate disability, severe disability, vegetative state, and death. Procedural limitations and lack of detail for each outcome category led to the development of the Glasgow Outcome Scale (GOS) Extended.[29] The GOS Extended scale is a widely used measure of global recovery after TBI. This 8-point scale provides greater detail on post-TBI functioning level than the original 5-point GOS by designating a lower and upper category for the good, moderate, and severe recovery levels. The GOS Extended provides a more structured approach to the interview process to accurately assess level of consciousness, functional independence, interpersonal relationships, and ability to work. The final score ranges from good recovery to death.[29] Functional and neurologic assessments are able to be performed by a trained assessor and guides the clinician in the need and individualization for rehabilitative care.

A comprehensive neuropsychological battery consisting of validated assessments may be required to further assess functional status after a TBI. Clinical evaluation is often necessary to determine an individual's ability to return to work and other previously held roles. A plethora of assessments exist, allowing for specific measures to be chosen based on concerns such as injury severity, location of injury, symptom presentation, and individual functional goals of survivors. Language, memory, attention, spatial ability, psychomotor speed, executive function, symptom status, and emotional status are commonly assessed domains. Assessments can be performed at various intervals to assess change in functioning over time. This process guides the clinician's evaluation of the patient's progress and therefore drives the potential therapies prescribed for a full outcome.

Special populations: the elderly patient with a traumatic brain injury   With the increased aging population projected in the United States, the impact of TBI on older adults has become an important public health issue. The elderly population is at an increased risk of TBI, higher mortality rates, and worse functional outcomes compared with younger patients.[30–32] The incidence of chronic subdural hematomas is expected to double by 2030.[33] Care in the postacute phase can be complex and requires a multidisciplinary effort between physicians, nurses, case managers, rehabilitation specialists, and personal care partners, such as a family member or friend.

Although older age is associated with higher mortality and worse functional outcome, the American College of Surgeons–Trauma Quality Improvement Program guidelines advises that age alone should not be considered a reason to withhold treatment for TBI.[34] Communication with the patient or care partner/family is essential to confirm the level of independence and function before the injury. A comprehensive health history is essential to establish baseline comorbidities, especially those that may affect neurologic function, such as preexisting dementia, stroke with motor or speech deficits, or hearing or vision deficits. These conditions have a significant influence over patient management across the continuum. Other comorbid conditions that require anticoagulation should be documented, because these medications may exacerbate the progression of TBI and delay healing. Reversal of these medications is a goal in early TBI management, and the timing of resuming these medications is often discussed after hospital discharge.

Postacute follow-up care is not standardized and varies widely across providers. Follow-up assessments generally consist of a neurologic examination that may include the GCS examination, assessment of cranial nerves, a fall risk assessment, and subjective reporting of any new or worsening symptoms as listed in the Post-Concussion Symptom Score.[35] The presence of a caregiver is helpful in verifying any deficits that may have existed before the injury.

The patient's medication list should be reviewed and updated accordingly with the patient or care partner. The education about the medication list is usually provided by the nurse. Preinjury polypharmacy is an independent predictor of mortality and may increase mortality risk by a factor of 2.3 times in this patient population.[36] Elderly patients are more likely to require anticoagulant medications, which are often withheld during the acute phase of care and may resume after verifying that the injury has resolved by review of radiographic imaging, and at the discretion of the neurosurgeon and the physician who initially recommended anticoagulation to treat the preexisting condition. Because elderly patients are more likely to have preexisting comorbidities, polypharmacy is a significant concern in clinical management, because this population is more likely to experience adverse side effects from multiple medications. The medication list should be evaluated with consideration of safety and effectiveness of prescribed treatments.[37]

Updated and current radiographic brain imaging should be reviewed to ensure that the lesion has resolved. Elderly patients are at risk for developing residual fluid collections and may often seem to be asymptomatic. A persistent fluid collection may not require treatment unless there is significant reaccumulation of fluid or the patient exhibits neurologic decline.[38]

Postacute Complications Associated with Severe Traumatic Brain Injury

Patients with severe TBI, especially those who have undergone a decompressive craniectomy, are at risk for several potential complications that may occur days to months after stabilization in the ICU or initial hospitalization. These complications have the potential to delay progress in cognitive function and may even be potentially life threatening. Clinicians in the postacute setting should educate care partners on the signs and symptoms that would prompt emergent neurosurgical management at discharge and should reinforce recommendations at postacute clinic follow-up visits.

CLINICAL IMPLICATIONS

The diagnosis of TBI many times has lifelong implications, whether the injury is mild, moderate, or severe. Specialized, evidenced-based care from the time of injury and on through rehabilitation is paramount in achieving the best patient outcomes. Mild TBI has been shown to have a delay in return to normal activities, with approximately 33% of these patients showing impairment at 3 months after the injury.[3] Stein and colleagues[39] have shown that the risk of posttraumatic stress disorder (PTSD) and/or major depressive disorder symptoms are present in 20% of cases of mild TBI at 3 months after an injury and in 21% at 6 months. Symptoms may develop in the hyperacute phase and education for the individual and family is paramount to avoid maladaptation to symptoms. A study by Seabury and colleagues[40] identified gaps in follow-up care of patients with a mild TBI discharged from the emergency room, with less than one-half self-reported as receiving TBI educational materials at discharge. Nurses, as advocates, would be ideal providers to promote this follow-up education. With increasing awareness of the signs and symptoms of concussion, it is becoming apparent that those patients with mild TBI fare better if meticulous acute care and long-term follow-up in clinic as well as referral to support systems (eg, support groups, psychology, occupational therapy, physical therapy) is provided to maintain an optimal quality of life.

Table 2
Common complications following a severe TBI

Complication	Risk Factors Related to TBI	Clinical Presentation	Diagnosis	Treatment
Cranial infections Subdural empyema	• After neurosurgical procedures	Fever Sinusitis Otitis Focal neurologic deficits Seizure activity Signs of increased ICP Decreasing LOC Headache Nuchal rigidity	CT MRI Lumbar puncture	Conservative treatment with antibiotics, symptom management Surgical treatment with burr hole drainage, craniotomy or craniectomy
Cranial infections Cerebral abscess	• Penetrating head trauma • Basilar skull fracture with associated CSF leak	Headache and nausea and/or vomiting Fever Seizure activity Focal neurologic deficits Altered mental status with nuchal rigidity	Elevated WBC Elevated ESR Blood cultures Common microorganisms: *Staphylococcus*, *Streptococcus*, and *Pneumococcus* CT with or without contrast MRI with or without contrast	Antibiotics Surgical drainage and/or excision (for lesions >2.5 cm) Steroids (to treat edema)
Cranial infections: infected bone flap	• Incidence ranges between 0.5% and 11.0%, with craniofacial and emergency surgeries carrying a greater risk of infection • Presence of other foreign bodies such as ICP monitors, EVDs, titanium plates	Fever Scalp tenderness Discharge from sinus tract Headache Nausea/vomiting Lethargy Fever Meningismus Periorbital Swelling Focal neurologic deficits	Clinical Presentation Culture of wound drainage, if present WBC ESR CRP Procalcitonin Skull radiograph CT MRI with and without contrast	Surgical revision Debridement and removal of infected bone flap, followed by delayed cranioplasty Antibiotics

(continued on next page)

Table 2
(continued)

Complication	Risk Factors Related to TBI	Clinical Presentation	Diagnosis	Treatment
Shunt infection	• Infection rate ranges from 8% to 15% • Greatest risk of infection occurs within the first 6 mo after placement	Can present as shunt failure: headache, nausea/vomiting, cranial nerve deficits, gait instability, and mental status change	CBC ESR CRP UA Blood cultures Shunt tap CT MRI Shunt series radiographs Shuntogram (if readily available and the patient is clinically stable)	Antibiotics CSF diversion with shunt externalization Conservative treatment with antibiotics (systemic and intraventricular) without externalization or removal of shunt (generally contraindicated in patients with *Staphylococcus aureus* infections) Removal of entire shunt system External ventricular drainage after removal of shunt system Repositioning distal catheter in another location such as the pleura, gallbladder, or atrium, in patients with intraabdominal infections or to allow for resolution of intraabdominal pseudocysts
Syndrome of the trephined	• Occurs in approximately 10% of postdecompressive craniectomy patients • "Sinking flap syndrome"	Characterized by neurologic dysfunction improved by cranioplasty Most common presenting symptom: motor weakness Followed by: cognitive deficits, decreased attention, memory	Clinical presentation A multifaceted approach is recommended that may include CT perfusion scan MRI EEG to rule out other conditions Radiographic findings of	Early cranioplasty

		impairment, executive function difficulties, language deficits, altered LOC, headache, psychosomatic disturbances, seizure activity, and cranial nerve deficits Symptoms can occur in a wide range from 3 d to 7 y after craniectomy, with average time of onset at approximately 5 mo after craniectomy	paradoxic herniation Deviation of midline structures	Conservative treatment (observation) if patient is asymptomatic Surgical removal with burr hole drainage or craniotomy
Subdural hygroma	• Occurs in 25%–50% patients after craniectomy	• Patients may be asymptomatic • Symptoms may correspond with a slowly developing subdural hematoma: headache that progressively becomes severe and persistent, drowsiness, confusion	CT scan with subdural fluid collection that is similar in appearance to a chronic subdural hematoma	
Posttraumatic epilepsy (late seizures)	• May occur early (within 7 d of injury) or late (onset is after 7 d after the injury) • Clinical signs may present in 12% of patients with severe TBI • Subclinical signs detected by EEG may be as high as 20%–25% • More common in older patients with TBI	Seizure activity	Radiographic imaging (CT or MRI) to rule out underlying cause in an acute onset seizure EEG	Antiepileptic medication

(continued on next page)

Table 2
(continued)

Complication	Risk Factors Related to TBI	Clinical Presentation	Diagnosis	Treatment

Shunt failure	• Proximal shunt occlusion
	• Distal shunt occlusion
	• Shunt infection
	• Failure rate is often highest within the first several months of initial shunt placement:
	  • 14% within the first month
	  • 40%–50% within the first year
	  • 49%–59% of all shunt patients will go on to require at least one shunt revision and often multiple shunt revisions
		Headache
		Nausea/vomiting
		Cranial nerve deficits
		Gait instability
		Mental status change
			Clinical Presentation
			CT
			MRI
			Shunt series radiographs
			Shuntogram (if readily available and the patient is clinically stable)
				Shunt exploration with possible revision

Abbreviations: CRP, C-reactive protein; CSF, cerebrospinal fluid; EEG, electroencephalogram; ESR, erythrocyte sedimentation rate; EVD, extraventricular drain; LOC, level of consciousness; UA, urinalysis; WBC, white blood cell count.

Patients with more severe TBI presentation will intuitively require more time to heal and will often need intensive TBI-specific rehabilitation and ongoing support. It is important for the clinician to advocate for entry into a system of care for these patients as unrecognized problems may worsen without regular follow-up and focused, individualized intervention (**Table 2**).

SUMMARY

Care and proper follow-up for the patient with a TBI, no matter how mild the injury, is needed. Concussive symptoms often do not appear at immediate presentation and the individual and caretaker need to be educated before discharge for mild TBI/concussive diagnoses. Across the spectrum of severity in TBI, the involvement of the nurse clinician is needed to advocate for continued care, if needed, and optimize and expedite realistic outcomes.

REFERENCES

1. Coronado VG, Xu L, Basavaraju SV, et al. Surveillance for traumatic brain injury-related deaths–United States, 1997-2007. MMWR Surveill Summ 2011; 60(5):1–32.
2. Bushnik T, Englander J, Wright J, et al. Traumatic brain injury with and without late posttraumatic seizures: what are the impacts in the post-acute phase: a NIDRR traumatic brain injury model systems study. J Head Trauma Rehabil 2012; 27(6):E36–44.
3. McMahon PJ, Hricik A, Yue JK, et al. Symptomatology and functional outcome in mild traumatic brain injury: results from the prospective TRACK-TBI study. J neurotrauma 2014;31(1):26–33.
4. van der Horn HJ, Spikman JM, Jacobs B, et al. Postconcussive complaints, anxiety, and depression related to vocational outcome in minor to severe traumatic brain injury. Arch Phys Med Rehabil 2013;94(5):867–74.
5. Gooden JR, Ponsford JL, Chariton JL, et al. The development and initial validation of a new tool to measure self-awareness of driving ability after brain injury. Aust Occup Ther J 2017;64(1):33–40.
6. The ATLS Subcommittee, American College of Surgeons' Committee on Trauma, and the International ATLS Working Group, ATLS® student manual. 9th edition. Chicago: American College of Surgeons; 2012.
7. Carney N, Totten AM, O'reilly C, et al. Guidelines for the management of severe traumatic brain injury. Neurosurgery 2017;80(1):6–15.
8. Torres A, Niederman MS, Chastre J, et al. International ERS/ESICM/ESCMID/ALAT guidelines for the management of hospital-acquired pneumonia and ventilator-associated pneumonia: guidelines for the management of hospital-acquired pneumonia (HAP)/ventilator-associated pneumonia (VAP) of the European Respiratory Society (ERS), European Society of Intensive Care Medicine (ESICM), European Society of Clinical Microbiology and Infectious Diseases (ESCMID) and Asociación Latinoamericana del Tórax (ALAT). Eur Respir J 2017;50(3):1700582.
9. Bouadma L, Sonneville R, Garrouste-Orgeas M, et al. Ventilator-associated events: prevalence, outcome, and relationship with ventilator-associated pneumonia. Crit Care Med 2015;43(9):1798–806.
10. Hendrickson CM, Howard BM, Kornblith LZ, et al. The acute respiratory distress syndrome following isolated severe traumatic brain injury. J Trauma Acute Care Surg 2016;80(6):989.

11. Narayan RK, Kishore PR, Becker DP, et al. Intracranial pressure: to monitor or not monitor? A review of our experience with severe head injury. J Neurosurg 1982; 56(5):650–9.

12. Chen H, Yuan F, Chen S-W, et al. Predicting posttraumatic hydrocephalus: derivation and validation of a risk scoring system based on clinical characteristics. Metab Brain Dis 2017;32(5):1427–35.

13. Jacobsson L, Westerberg M, Lexell J. Health-related quality-of-life and life satisfaction 6–15 years after traumatic brain injuries in northern Sweden. Brain Inj 2010;24(9):1075–86.

14. Rogers S, Richards KC, Davidson M, et al. Description of the moderate brain injured patient and predictors of discharge to rehabilitation. Arch Phys Med Rehabil 2015;96(2):276–82.

15. Harrison AL, Hunter EG, Thomas H, et al. Living with traumatic brain injury in a rural setting: supports and barriers across the continuum of care. Disabil Rehabil 2017;39(20):2071–80.

16. Zarshenas S, Tam L, Colantonio A, et al. Predictors of discharge destination from acute care in patients with traumatic brain injury. BMJ Open 2017;7(8):e016694.

17. Batchelor JS, Grayson A. A meta-analysis to determine the effect of anticoagulation on mortality in patients with blunt head trauma. Br J Neurosurg 2012;26(4): 525–30.

18. Albrecht JS, Liu X, Baumgarten M, et al. Benefits and risks of anticoagulation resumption following traumatic brain injury. JAMA Intern Med 2014;174(8): 1244–51.

19. Frey LC. Epidemiology of posttraumatic epilepsy: a critical review. Epilepsia 2003;44:11–7.

20. Chartrain AG, Yaeger K, Feng R, et al. Antiepileptics for post-traumatic seizure prophylaxis after traumatic brain injury. Curr Pharm Des 2017;23(42):6428–41.

21. Temkin NR, Dikmen SS, Wilensky AJ, et al. A randomized, double-blind study of phenytoin for the prevention of post-traumatic seizures. N Engl J Med 1990; 323(8):497–502.

22. Szaflarski JP, Sangha KS, Lindsell CJ, et al. Prospective, randomized, single-blinded comparative trial of intravenous levetiracetam versus phenytoin for seizure prophylaxis. Neurocrit Care 2010;12(2):165–72.

23. Inaba K, Menaker J, Branco BC, et al. A prospective multicenter comparison of levetiracetam versus phenytoin for early posttraumatic seizure prophylaxis. J Trauma Acute Care Surg 2013;74(3):766–73.

24. Gironda RJ, Clark ME, Ruff RL, et al. Traumatic brain injury, polytrauma, and pain: challenges and treatment strategies for the polytrauma rehabilitation. Rehabil Psychol 2009;54(3):247.

25. Derogatis LR. BSI, brief symptom inventory: administration, scoring and procedures manual 1993. Google Scholar.

26. Meachen S-J, Hanks RA, Millis SR, et al. The reliability and validity of the brief symptom inventory– 18 in persons with traumatic brain injury. Arch Phys Med Rehabil 2008;89(5):958–65.

27. Iverson GL, Lovell MR, Collins MW. Interpreting change on ImPact following sport concussion. Clin Neuropsychol 2003;17:460–7.

28. Jennett B, Bond MR. Assessment of outcome after severe brain damage. Lancet 1975;1:480–4.

29. Wilson JL, Pettigrew LE, Teasdale GM. Structured interviews for the Glasgow Outcome Scale and the extended Glasgow Outcome Scale: guidelines for their use. J Neurotrauma 1998;15(8):573–85.

30. Susman M, DiRusso SM, Sullivan T, et al. Traumatic brain injury in the elderly: increased mortality and worse functional outcome at discharge despite lower injury severity. J Trauma Acute Care Surg 2002;53(2):219–24.
31. Fletcher AE, Khalid S, Mallonee S. The epidemiology of severe traumatic brain injury among persons 65 years of age and older in Oklahoma, 1992–2003. Brain Inj 2007;21(7):691–9.
32. Haring RS, Narang K, Canner JK, et al. Traumatic brain injury in the elderly: morbidity and mortality trends and risk factors. J Surg Res 2015;195(1):1–9.
33. Soleman J, Nocera F, Mariani L. The conservative and pharmacological management of chronic subdural haematoma. Swiss Med Wkly 2017;147:w14398.
34. Surgeons ACo. ACS TQIP geriatric trauma management guidelines. Trauma quality improvement Program (TQIP). Available at: www.facs.org/~/media/files/quality%20programs/trauma/tqip/geriatric%20guide%20tqip.ashx. Accessed February 26, 2019.
35. Joyce AS, Labella CR, Carl RL, et al. The post-concussion symptom scale: utility of a three-factor structure. Med Sci Sports Exerc 2015;47(6):1119–23.
36. Catapano JS, Chapman AJ, Horner LP, et al. Pre-injury polypharmacy predicts mortality in isolated severe traumatic brain injury patients. Am J Surg 2017; 213(6):1104–8.
37. Cosano G, Giangreco M, Ussai S, et al. Polypharmacy and the use of medications in inpatients with acquired brain injury during post-acute rehabilitation: a cross-sectional study. Brain Inj 2016;30(3):353–62.
38. Mehta V, Harward SC, Sankey EW, et al. Evidence based diagnosis and management of chronic subdural hematoma: a review of the literature. J Clin Neurosci 2018;50:7–15.
39. Stein MB, Jain S, Giacino JT, et al. Risk of posttraumatic stress disorder and major depression in civilian patients after mild traumatic brain injury: a TRACK-TBI study. JAMA Psychiatry 2019;76(3):249–58.
40. Seabury SA, Gaudette E, Goldman DP, et al. Assessment of follow-up care after emergency department presentation for mild traumatic brain injury and concussion: results from the TRACK-TBI study. JAMA Netw Open 2018;1(1):e180210.

The Projected Care Trajectory for Persons with Epilepsy

Wendy R. Miller, PhD, RN, CNS, CCRN

KEYWORDS

- Epilepsy • Seizures • Self-management • Chronic disease • Neuroscience nursing

KEY POINTS

- Epilepsy is a common, chronic neurologic disease that requires complex medical management, as well as self-management.
- People with epilepsy often require specialized medical care from a neurologist or epileptologist. A shortage of these types of providers inhibits the ability of patients with epilepsy to receive timely specialized care.
- People with epilepsy commonly experience psychiatric comorbidities, which require treatment by a neuropsychologist, psychologist, or psychiatrist.
- Optimal care of persons with epilepsy and their families relies on integrated care and epilepsy self-management support.

INTRODUCTION

The fourth most common neurologic disease in the world, epilepsy is a brain disease that affects people of all ages and is characterized by the occurrence of unprovoked seizures and other epilepsy-related health problems. One out of every 26 people is diagnosed with epilepsy at some point in their lifetimes, and there are currently 3.4 million Americans living with epilepsy, 3 million of whom are adults.[1] Epilepsy is a spectrum condition, with a wide range of severity affecting those with the disease.[1] The hallmark of epilepsy is a seizure, which is a sudden surge of electrical activity in the brain. Seizures affect the way a person appears or acts for a short period of time, and are classified according to a system that is descriptive of the area of origin of the seizure; whether a person's awareness is affected; and whether the seizure involves other symptoms, such as movement. Thus, a seizure can be focal (affecting 1 part of the brain) or generalized (affecting more than 1 part of the brain) in onset, and associated with alteration/no alteration in awareness and movement/no movement.

Disclosure: The author has nothing to disclose.
Department of Community Health Systems, Indiana University School of Nursing, 600 Barnhill Drive, Indianapolis, IN 46202, USA
E-mail address: wrtruebl@iu.edu

The International League Against Epilepsy[2] provides the most up-to-date seizure classification systems. The postictal period, the recovery period following a seizure, is characterized by symptoms such as fatigue, confusion, anxiety, fear, and problems communicating verbally or via writing, and may last hours or days.[1]

At present, there is no cure for epilepsy; it is a chronic disease that is managed throughout the person's life. Persons with epilepsy (PWEs) are at high risk for experiencing psychiatric comorbidities, such as mood, anxiety, and psychotic disorders, and also face a myriad of social functioning problems.[3] Epilepsy can also be fatal, via direct epilepsy-related causes (sudden, unexpected death in epilepsy [SUDEP]), injury from a seizure, or status epilepticus (continuous seizure activity).[1] Being diagnosed and living with epilepsy is thus complex, and has been described by patients as completely life altering.[4] From the onset of symptoms and diagnosis of epilepsy to management of the disease throughout the lifespan, the patients and their family members undergo many transitions. Health care professionals, and especially nurses and advanced practice nurses, are instrumental in supporting PWEs and their families through these transitions in pursuit of desirable levels of disease management and quality of life, as well as optimal levels of functioning. That is, nurses are uniquely situated to support PWEs in improving their perceived health as defined by nursing: a composite evaluation of both illness and wellness experiences (how patients function and feel physically and mentally) despite the presence of disease.[5]

EPILEPSY DIAGNOSIS PROCESS

The experience of a seizure does not automatically lead to a diagnosis of epilepsy; seizures that have a known, reversible cause (eg, hypoglycemia) are not associated with epilepsy. In order to qualify for an epilepsy diagnosis, a person must meet at least 1 of the following criteria: (1) experience of at least 2 unprovoked seizures occurring more than 24 hours apart; (2) experience of 1 unprovoked seizure and a probability of further seizures similar to the general recurrence risk (60%) after 2 unprovoked seizures, occurring over the next 10 years; or (3) diagnosis of an epilepsy syndrome.[6] New-onset epilepsy can occur at any point in the lifespan, with peak occurrence in young children and older adults.[1]

A first seizure, or first seizure that has resulted in seeking medical attention, regardless of type, is an extremely fear-inducing experience for patients and family members, and is also associated with feelings of shame, embarrassment, and uncertainty.[1] Patients experiencing generalized, impaired-awareness seizures with motor involvement (previously known as grand mal and tonic-clonic seizures) most commonly present to the emergency department (ED) for initial treatment. Patients who experience less well-known and more subtle types of seizures (focal seizures with or without impaired awareness or motor involvement, previously known as simple/complex seizures, or generalized seizures with impaired awareness but no motor involvement, previously known as absence seizures) are more likely to present to a primary care provider (PCP) with their symptoms, and are also more likely to attribute their seizure-related symptoms to something else (eg, inattention in children or forgetfulness in older adults).[7,8] Anyone presenting with a first seizure undergoes a multitude of diagnostic tests. The patients have any reversible cause (eg, hypoglycemia) ruled out via laboratory studies, followed by imaging and, often, an electroencephalogram (EEG). For two-thirds of PWEs, the cause is unknown. In the remaining third, the most common causes are stroke, tumor, infection, traumatic brain injury (TBI), anoxic brain injury, and genetic disorders.[9,10]

Although most people who develop epilepsy do so suddenly in either childhood or adulthood without any clear cause, adults and older adults develop epilepsy related to 2 main causes: TBI and stroke. Identified by the Centers for Disease Control and Prevention (CDC) as a public health issue,[11] TBI is a significant cause of epilepsy. Post-traumatic epilepsy occurs in up to 53% of TBIs, with risk factors including TBI severity, presence of intracranial bleeding, and early experience of seizures after TBI.[12] In older adults, who are the population in which new-onset epilepsy is most prevalent, stroke is the most common cause of epilepsy.[13] Older adults living in long-term care facilities have a 7-fold increase in the prevalence of epilepsy compared with community-dwelling older adults, and most of these instances are related to stroke.[14] Thus, many people newly diagnosed with epilepsy must adapt to this chronic disease in the midst of other health-related events; the management of epilepsy in conjunction with other health problems is especially difficult for PWEs and their family caregivers.[7,8]

Note that, for many patients newly diagnosed with epilepsy, the journey to an accurate diagnosis has not been swift. Especially for those experiencing seizures that lack motor involvement, achieving an appropriate diagnosis of epilepsy can take years. In older adults, the length of time from first seizure to diagnosis has been recorded as up to 7 years.[8] Thus, at the time of diagnosis, PWEs can be exhausted and frustrated with the health care system. The Institute of Medicine, in its report on epilepsy,[15] noted the need to better educate PCPs and ED providers, as well as the public, on the many different kinds of seizures that people can experience. In 2016, The Epilepsy Foundation launched a campaign called #ShareMySeizure, in which PWEs shared and discussed their nonmovement seizures; video of participants having these seizures was included in the campaign.[16] Public and provider awareness that seizures come in many forms other than generalized impaired awareness with movement (tonic-clonic) is imperative to reducing diagnosis times in PWEs.

MEDICAL MANAGEMENT OF EPILEPSY

Once an epilepsy diagnosis has been made, the patient and family must adapt to the presence of a chronic, potentially life-threatening disease. Patients presenting with a first seizure may receive epilepsy care from a PCP, but often they transition to the care of a specialist. However, the United States currently has a significant shortage of neurologists.[17–19] Patients diagnosed with epilepsy in the ED are often sent home on an antiseizure drug (ASD) and receive a referral to a neurologist, which, in most parts of the country, can be associated with a wait of several months. Those presenting to a PCP not willing or able to manage the epilepsy must also wait many months to be evaluated by a neurologist. The time between diagnosis and entry to care with a specialist, termed the waiting period, is extremely trying for PWEs and their families, and is associated with unnecessary ED visits in the case of subsequent seizures.[1] PWEs report that the information given to them on diagnosis is not comprehensive and that they are unprepared for how to manage the condition, ASDs and their side effects, and daily life in the presence of new restrictions, such as inability to drive. They are also unsure of when a seizure is considered an emergency and when it is not.[4,8,20] This period of time from diagnosis to specialized evaluation and treatment is particularly challenging for both PWEs and their families, and has been described by PWEs as the "black hole period" as the newness of the disease settles in, along with changes in independence and the uncertainty of seizure occurrence.[4] PWEs and their family members have also reported being sent home to wait on a neurologist without even understanding what epilepsy is[21]; this lack of information is extremely dangerous, because it can affect medication and activity restriction adherence. There is a need for supportive interventions during this key and at-risk transition period, beginning with discharge from the ED/PCP. Discharge planning that is focused on how to manage seizures at home, when an ambulance should be called, and connection with resources such as a case manager or social worker should be prioritized.[15]

TRANSITION FROM NEUROLOGIST TO EPILEPTOLOGIST

Most PWEs (~70%) can have their epilepsy managed by a general neurologist via the use of ASDs (preferably a single ASD).[15] However, if a person's seizures and side effects have not been controlled after 1 year overseen by a neurologist, the patient should be referred to a specialized epilepsy center to be evaluated and treated by an epileptologist, a neurologist who specializes and has undergone extensive training in epilepsy treatment.[15] In addition to epileptologists, epilepsy centers have psychologists/psychiatrists, pharmacists, nurse-clinicians, nurse educators, dieticians, and other health care professionals who specialize in PWEs and work as a team to provide optimal epilepsy care.[22] Both level 3 and level 4 epilepsy centers can provide specialized epilepsy care, with level 4 centers offering more advanced surgical treatments. However, in the United States, there is a shortage of epileptologists, resulting in long wait times, and many people living with epilepsy are hundreds of miles away from the nearest specialized epilepsy center. For example, there are no epilepsy centers in either North or South Dakota.[23] Thus, to ensure a more timely transition to specialized epilepsy care when needed, referrals to epilepsy centers should be made as early as possible. PWEs and their families should be encouraged to advocate for specialty referral when it is needed. The Epilepsy Foundation of America encourages patients and family members to know the criteria for referral and to address it candidly with their neurologists.[22] If referral to a specialized epilepsy center is not made when it is appropriate to do so, the patient is put in danger because of the potential for an inaccurate diagnosis (eg, the patient does not have epilepsy but is being treated for it); experience of seizures, which increases the person's risk for SUDEP; and experience of side effects, which affect overall functioning, relationships, and quality of life. Of the roughly 30% of PWEs who do not achieve seizure and side effect control under the care of a neurologist, less than one-fourth are evaluated and treated at a level 3 or 4 epilepsy center.[15]

When PWEs are referred to an epilepsy center, the PWEs and their family members enter another waiting period, which is approximately 4 weeks in the United States.[23] If the epilepsy center, most of which are associated with academic medical centers in urban areas, is far from the PWE's home, the patient and family must arrange for travel and lodging near the center. Once the PWE is seen in the epilepsy clinic, the patient and family encounter a different approach to epilepsy treatment. First, epileptologists often elect to observe patients in an epilepsy monitoring unit (EMU), a specialized inpatient unit in which PWEs can be observed over time using specialized diagnostics. The length of stay in the EMU ranges from approximately 4 to 7 days, and is used for event characterization, medication adjustment, or presurgical evaluation. While in the EMU, the PWEs are connected to long-term video EEG monitoring, and medications may be withdrawn in order to precipitate a seizure that can be captured during the monitoring. Because of the intentional provocation of seizures and long length of stay, the EMU can be extremely stressful for both PWEs and their family members.[24] Providing PWEs and family members with clear education regarding the reasoning for ASD withdrawal and activity restriction within the EMU has been shown to increase comfort of PWEs and family members in this care setting, and PWEs found presence of family in the EMU to be helpful as well.[24] There is a need to develop support structures for family members of PWEs in the EMU, because leaving home/work responsibilities for an extended period of time is not always feasible, and waiting for a loved one to have a seizure is stressful.

Once a PWE has been evaluated in an EMU, the epileptologist and team can consider the best course of action, but have many more options available than those of a general neurologist: medications that have not yet been tried; device implantation, such as a vagus nerve stimulator; or several types of brain surgery. In some cases, the ketogenic diet, under the direction of a specially trained dietician, may be recommended as well. The PWE and family members may feel overwhelmed when faced with these new treatments, particularly surgery, which involves extensive presurgical screening and leads to seizure freedom in two-thirds of cases. Epilepsy clinics, using social workers, nurses, advanced practice nurses, psychiatrists, and other specialists, are well equipped to counsel PWEs and family members about treatment decisions while taking into account each person's overall health and functioning. Most (66.4%) PWEs who enter an epilepsy clinic for care remain in that or a similar clinic for epilepsy treatment. The remaining PWEs are managed medically by their referring providers.[15]

REFERRAL TO MENTAL HEALTH PROVIDERS

PWEs are at high risk for psychiatric comorbidities, and are 2 to 3 times more likely to experience mood disorders, depression, anxiety, suicide, and psychosis compared with people without epilepsy. PWEs are also more likely to be socially isolated, less likely to be employed, and more likely to experience relationship problems. Therefore, referral to a mental health provider is often integral to the care of PWEs.[3] The mental health care provider to whom a PWE is referred depends on that person's specific comorbidities and symptoms; for example, neuropsychiatric problems involving cognition, behavior, attention, and learning should be assessed and treated by a neuropsychologist. Psychologists or psychiatrists are integral to assessing and managing PWEs' mental health conditions and symptoms, such as depression and anxiety. Many PWEs benefit from both neuropsychological and psychological/psychiatric evaluation and treatment. PWEs are especially likely to develop psychiatric comorbidities in the first year following diagnosis, making astute evaluation for these symptoms vital.[25]

However, many PWEs do not receive the psychiatric/mental health care needed because of underreporting by patients, who may fear stigma or not be aware of the need to address psychiatric comorbidities, and also because some providers are under the impression that psychiatric medications, such as antidepressants, lower the seizure threshold in PWEs. Psychotropic drugs should be used cautiously in PWEs, but should not be withheld when needed.[26] Given the high incidence of psychiatric comorbidities in PWEs, it is important for psychiatric care to be integrated into the care of PWEs. Level 3 and 4 epilepsy centers typically have neuropsychologists, psychologists, and psychiatrists on staff who specialize in treating PWEs. For PWEs managed by PCPs or neurologists, a referral to a mental health provider may take longer or never occur. Untreated psychiatric comorbidities can be devastating. Because of the potential for psychiatric referrals not occurring for PWEs outside of epilepsy centers, the Epilepsy Foundation encourages PWEs and their families to report psychiatric symptoms to their providers and to advocate for referral.[27] Ideally, PWEs and their family members are educated about the likely onset of psychiatric symptoms and comorbidities at the time of epilepsy diagnosis.

TRANSITION FROM PEDIATRIC TO ADULT EPILEPSY CARE

One of the most significant transitions in care experienced by children with epilepsy, as well as their parents and other family members, is the transition from pediatric to adult epilepsy care. It is important that children with epilepsy and their families experience a true transition, as opposed to transfer, of care during late adolescence or early adulthood. This transition should be a structured process based on planning, preparation, and involvement of skilled epilepsy practitioners. The patient and parents/other family members should be carefully prepared for the transition in care, rather than handed off to the adult model of care once the patient reaches 18 years of age.[28]

Parents of children with epilepsy are heavily involved in the transition to adult epilepsy management. Up until the point of transition, parents have overseen and directed physician and other provider visits, and pediatric medical care is more family centered. Once a PWE reaches the adult care setting, care is focused on the individual, and the individual is more likely to attend provider visits alone. This lack of control faced by parents of young adult PWEs is difficult for parents, and it is important to include them throughout the transition process. Transition clinics, in which pediatric and adult epilepsy providers practice, have been shown to be helpful in easing the transition between pediatric and adult epilepsy management.[28]

There is evidence that children with epilepsy who become adult PWEs have poorer social outcomes than those without the disease. Compared with adults without epilepsy, adults who have had epilepsy since childhood have problems obtaining employment, and are less likely to be married or partnered, to participate in a social life, and to have hobbies outside of work and family.[28] This risk for poor outcomes in this population underscores the importance of proper transition of epilepsy care from pediatric, which is more overseen by parents and other family members, to adult, which is more independent. To address the need for proper pediatric-to-adult transition in PWE, the Ontario Epilepsy Implementation Task Force recently published evidence-based guidelines for a smooth and effective transition. The task force recommends a 7-part transition process: introduce the concept of transition when the patient is between ages 12 and 15 years; explore financial, legal, and community support available when the patient is between ages 12 and 17 years; determine transition readiness of patients and their parents when the patient is between ages 16 and 17 years; identify and address risk factors for unsuccessful transition when the patient is between ages 12 and 19 years (risk factors differ depending on presence or absence of intellectual disability); reevaluate the epilepsy diagnosis when the patient is between ages 16 and 17 years; identify obstacles for continuation of treatment of drug-resistant epilepsies when the patient is between ages 16 and 17 years; and prepare the pediatric discharge packet when the patient is between ages 17 and 18 years. The pediatric discharge packet should include psychosocial screening results; transition readiness questionnaires; epilepsy history form; seizure emergency plan; goals of care; and community, social, and financial support.[29]

LONG-TERM SELF-MANAGEMENT OF EPILEPSY

At the onset of epilepsy, PWEs and their families face a major transition: being charged with managing a new chronic disease. Patients and their family members often manage epilepsy in the community (at home) in collaboration with epilepsy providers. More severe forms of epilepsy may require family members to rely on home health care or skilled nursing facilities. Epilepsy self-management (ESM) is an important factor in the overall management of epilepsy. As part of its 2012 report on epilepsy, the

Institute of Medicine[15] noted that achievement of positive outcomes in epilepsy depends on patients' involvement in managing the disease (self-management).

ESM has been defined and measured in multiple ways. Definitions range from describing behaviors in which PWEs engage to maintain adherence treatments,[30] ESM practices engaged by PWEs in 5 different areas (medication, information, safety, seizure, and lifestyle management),[31] to ESM being a complex process involving behaviors at multiple levels of a person's environment.[32] A holistic and systems-level definition of ESM is offered by Miller and colleagues,[32(p161)] who espouse ESM, and chronic disease self-management in general, as "a fluid, iterative process during which patients incorporate multidimensional strategies that meet their self-identified needs to cope with chronic disease within the context of their daily living. Strategies are multidimensional because they require the individual to incorporate intrapersonal, interpersonal, and environmental systems to maximize wellness. Successful management of both functioning in day-to-day life along with management of chronic illness requires the individual to continually monitor health and functional status and take appropriate actions during acute phases." Most published definitions of ESM have 1 common theme: it involves the day-to-day process through which PWEs, their families, friends, and others in their environment manage life in the context of having epilepsy.

Patients with epilepsy and their family members report feeling unprepared for ESM.[32] Although PWEs are tasked with navigating daily life with a disease that affects mood, memory, attention, and independence, is associated with unpredictable seizures, and is also highly stigmatized, caregivers and siblings of PWEs report lower quality of life and increased stress related to their family member's epilepsy. Epilepsy is also a major financial burden for families, related to expensive medical care or adult PWEs' inability to work consistently.[33,34] Recent research also indicates that adult PWEs experience significant intimate relationship problems.[35] That is, epilepsy and day-to-day ESM affects an entire family, whether the PWE is an adult or a child. Thus, preparation of PWEs and their family members or others involved in their ESM to effectively self-manage is paramount in achieving desirable epilepsy outcomes, including lower health care resource use and hospital admissions. Some ESM interventions are available via the Managing Epilepsy Well Network. These interventions include Web Epilepsy Awareness Support and Education (WebEASE), Home Based Self-management and Cognitive Training Changes Lives (HOBSCOTCH), Program for Active Consumer Engagement in Self-management (PACES in Epilepsy), Program to Encourage Active Rewarding Lives (PEARLS), and Using Practice and Learning to Increase Favorable Thoughts (UPLIFT for Epilepsy) (Managing Epilepsy Well).[36] A current priority in epilepsy research is the design and testing of patient-centered, sustainable, and scalable interventions that can be consumed by all PWEs in order to improve their ESM.[15] These types of interventions help ensure stable, successful transitions from epilepsy diagnosis to community-based ESM that is successful in minimizing exacerbations (seizures or medication side effects) as well as improving the perceived health of both PWEs and their families.

PWEs with certain risk factors are at increased risk for poor ESM. Social status, defined as a person's standing in society and comprising factors such as level of employment, education, insurance coverage, and income, has been shown to influence epilepsy-related outcomes. Researchers have found that lack of employment or underemployment, lower levels of education, poor or no insurance coverage, lower income, and living in a high-crime area are associated with more frequent use of emergency rooms by PWEs for epilepsy-related events, and with uncontrolled seizures,[37–39] which may indicate that people of lower social status are not able to

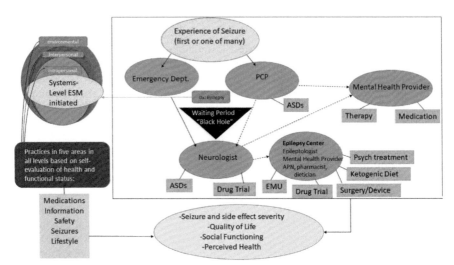

Fig. 1. Transitions that occur for people with epilepsy. APN, advanced practice nurse; Dx, diagnosis.

self-manage as well as those with higher levels of social status. It is thus important to consider and address each individual PWE's characteristics that impede or enhance the ability to engage in effective ESM.

SUMMARY

Epilepsy is a common neurologic condition that requires complex medical management and self-management. **Fig. 1** shows some key care transitions that occur for PWEs. Once a first seizure (or first seizure that requires medical attention) occurs, PWEs are typically diagnosed with epilepsy/seizures and referred to a specialist for care, which lands them and their families in the so-called black-hole waiting period. PWEs have their epilepsy managed by a PCP, neurologist, or an epilepsy-specific team, including an epileptologist, at an epilepsy center. Care provided at epilepsy centers is more integrated, with psychiatric, advanced practice nurse, pharmacy, and dietary care specific to epilepsy all available, and so focus on timely referrals for PWEs being treated outside of epilepsy centers should be prioritized to avoid delays and to support more comprehensive care. General neurologists or PCPs are typically able to prescribe ASDs for PWEs and can manage those patients who respond quickly without the presence of significant side effects. However, neurologists or PCPs must be aware that, even with the achievement of seizure control with few to no side effects, PWEs are at risk for psychiatric comorbidities that may necessitate treatment via a referral. If a PWE being managed by a neurologist or PCP is not well-controlled with ASDs (both in seizure frequency/severity and side effects), the provider should refer the patient to an epilepsy center. The shortage of neurologists, epileptologists, and epilepsy centers complicates and slows transitions of care for PWEs. Nurses, whether caring for PWEs in the ED, outpatient setting, or acute care setting, should educate patient and family members regarding the potential need for specialty and/or mental health care given an epilepsy diagnosis. As epilepsy researchers and clinicians continue to better integrate the care for PWEs and meet the demand for patients needing epilepsy care, PWEs and their families must advocate for appropriate care transitions, including those related to pediatric to adult epilepsy care, when appropriate. The transitions listed in **Fig. 1** can be discussed with both providers and PWEs and their family members on epilepsy diagnosis to help ensure that PWEs and their family members are provided with the most comprehensive care possible as expeditiously as possible.

All PWEs, as well as their family members and/or friends, are involved in ESM. Effective chronic disease self-management, including that in epilepsy, is a learned skill that takes time, support, and opportunities for skill building. When someone is diagnosed with epilepsy, that person and the entire family must begin learning to engage in optimal ESM, which is a daunting task, especially in the case of a stigmatized, less-well-known disease such as epilepsy. The discharge and ongoing support needed by PWEs and their family members to become effective self-managers cannot be overstated. Nurses encountering PWEs and their families, regardless of care setting, can direct patients and family members to existing ESM interventions, as well as epilepsy.com, the Epilepsy Foundation's Web site, which is geared toward helping people manage epilepsy.

NURSING IMPLICATIONS

Nurses, who interact with patients, family members, and advanced providers, are well situated to educate providers, PWEs, and family members about appropriate and optimal transitions in care for PWEs, and to provide PWEs and family members with ESM resources that will bolster their ESM skills. At each stage of transition for PWEs and care partners, nurses can serve a unique role in facilitating transitions and optimal outcomes. The nurse's advocacy role, characterized by empathy with and protection of patients,[40] should be present throughout all transition phases for PWEs and their families. In the initial epilepsy diagnosis process, whether occurring in an ED or outpatient setting, nurses can ensure that each patient is treated holistically, with thorough but understandable explanations of diagnosis procedures provided to the patient and family members. In this advocacy role, nurses can be especially impactful in the transition to specialized care. As described earlier, this stage can be frustrating for patients and care partners, and they are particularly vulnerable to seizures and unnecessary ED visits during this time. Nurses should develop and advocate for the use of clear, concise, and accurate discharge education for patients newly diagnosed with epilepsy/seizures. The focus of this education should be on preparing patients and family members to reduce seizure risk and promote safety in the interim between diagnosis and entry to care. Likewise, nurses who interact with PWEs who are receiving care from a PCP or neurologist should ensure that patients and care partners are aware of the criteria for referral to an epilepsy center, as well as to mental health providers. In addition, nurses who interact with patients in the chronic stages of their epilepsy, in which they and their family members are engaging in self-management, should provide access, digitally or in print depending on patient/family preferences, to the various ESM resources that exist regarding epilepsy. In each transition phase, the nurses' awareness of the major obstacles and desired outcomes should guide their advocacy activities. In most cases, providing patients and their family members with information that will help them make informed health-related decisions and provide access to skill-building resources is most helpful to patients and families.

REFERENCES

1. America EFo. About epilepsy and seizures. 2018. Available at: https://www.epilepsy.com/learn/professionals/about-epilepsy-seizures. Accessed December 5, 2018.

2. Epilepsy ILA. Definition and classification. 2017. Available at: https://www.ilae.org/guidelines/definition-and-classification. Accessed December 5, 2018.

3. Josephson CB, Jette N. Psychiatric comorbidities in epilepsy. Int Rev Psychiatry 2017;29(5):409–24.

4. Unger WR, Buelow JM. Hybrid concept analysis of self-management in adults newly diagnosed with epilepsy. Epilepsy Behav 2009;14(1):89–95.

5. Lyon B. Getting back on track: nursing's autonomous scope of practice. St Louis (MO): Mosby; 1990.

6. Epilepsy ILA. The 2014 definition of epilepsy: a Perspective for patients and caregivers. 2014. Available at: https://www.ilae.org/guidelines/definition-and-classification/the-2014-definition-of-epilepsy-a-perspective-for-patients-and-caregivers. Accessed December 5, 2018.

7. Miller WR, Bakas T, Buelow JM. Problems, needs, and useful strategies in older adults self-managing epilepsy: Implications for patient education and future intervention programs. Epilepsy Behav 2014;31:25–30.

8. Miller WR, Buelow JM, Bakas T. Older adults and new-onset epilepsy: experiences with diagnosis. J Neurosci Nurs 2014;46(1):2–10.

9. Prevention CfDCa. Frequently Asked Questions about epilepsy. 2018. Available at: https://www.cdc.gov/epilepsy/about/faq.htm. Accessed December 5, 2018.

10. Elger CE, Hoppe C. Diagnostic challenges in epilepsy: seizure under-reporting and seizure detection. Lancet Neurol 2018;17(3):279–88.

11. Prevention CfDCa. TBIs and Injuries. 2018. Available at: https://www.cdc.gov/features/traumatic-brain-injury/index.html. Accessed December 5, 2018.

12. Verellen RM, Cavazos JE. Post-traumatic epilepsy: an overview. Therapy 2010;7(5):527–31.

13. Liu S, Yu W, Lu Y. The causes of new-onset epilepsy and seizures in the elderly. Neuropsychiatr Dis Treat 2016;12:1425–34.

14. Birnbaum AK, Leppik IE, Svensden K, et al. Prevalence of epilepsy/seizures as a comorbidity of neurologic disorders in nursing homes. Neurology 2017;88(8):7.

15. England MJ, Liverman CT, Schultz AM, et al. Epilepsy across the spectrum: promoting health and understanding. A summary of the Institute of Medicine report. Epilepsy Behav 2012;25(2):266–76.

16. America EFo. Share My seizure. 2016. Available at: https://www.epilepsy.com/make-difference/public-awareness/sharemyseizure. Accessed December 5, 2018.

17. How to cope with the neurologist shortage. Harv Health Lett 2013;38(9):8.

18. Anderson H, Rydell CM. Neurologist shortage "critical". Minn Med 2012;95(1):6.

19. Burton A. How do we fix the shortage of neurologists? Lancet Neurol 2018;17(6):2.

20. Long L, Reeves AL, Moore JG, et al. An assessment of epilepsy patients' knowledge of their disorder. Epilepsia 2000;41(6):4.

21. Mameniskiene R, Sakalauskaite-Juodeikiene E, Budrys V. People with epilepsy lack knowledge about their disease. Epilepsy Behav 2015;46:5.

22. America EFo. What is an epileptologist and who needs one?. 2013. Available at: https://www.epilepsy.com/article/2013/1/what-epileptologist-and-who-needs-one. Accessed December 5, 2018.

23. Centers NAoE. National association of epilepsy centers. 2018. Available at: https://www.naec-epilepsy.org/. Accessed December 5, 2018.

24. Egger-Rainer A, Trinka E, Hofler J, et al. Epilepsy monitoring - The patients' views: a qualitative study based on Kolcaba's Comfort Theory. Epilepsy Behav 2017;68:208–15.

25. Chang HJ, Liao CC, Hu CJ, et al. Psychiatric disorders after epilepsy diagnosis: a population-based retrospective cohort study. PLoS One 2013;8(4):e59999.
26. Puvvada SC, Kommisetti S, Reddy A. Managing psychiatric illness in patients with epilepsy. Curr Psychiatry 2014;13(5):8.
27. America EFo. Overview of depression. 2018. Available at: https://www.epilepsy.com/living-epilepsy/healthy-living/emotional-health/overview-depression. Accessed December 5, 2018.
28. Rajendran S, Iyer A. Epilepsy: addressing the transition from pediatric to adult care. Adolesc Health Med Ther 2016;7:77–87.
29. Andrade DM, Bassett AS, Bercovici E, et al. Epilepsy: Transition from pediatric to adult care. Recommendations of the Ontario epilepsy implementation task force. Epilepsia 2017;58(9):1502–17.
30. McAuley JW, McFadden LS, Elliott JO, et al. An evaluation of self-management behaviors and medication adherence in patients with epilepsy. Epilepsy Behav 2008;13(4):637–41.
31. Dilorio C, Shafer PO, Letz R, et al. Behavioral, social, and affective factors associated with self-efficacy for self-management among people with epilepsy. Epilepsy Behav 2006;9:5.
32. Miller WR, Lasiter S, Bartlett Ellis R, et al. Chronic disease self-management: a hybrid concept analysis. Nurs Outlook 2015;63(2):154–61.
33. Ostendorf AP, Gedela S. Effect of epilepsy on families, communities, and society. Semin Pediatr Neurol 2017;24(4):340–7.
34. Mohamed MA, Hassan MA, Mohamed MF. Effect of epilepsy on the quality of life of children and their family caregivers. J Nurs Health Sci 2018;7(5):8.
35. Miller WR, Gesselman AN, Garcia JR, et al. Epilepsy-related romantic and sexual relationship problems and concerns: Indications from Internet message boards. Epilepsy Behav 2017;74:149–53.
36. Network MEW. Managing epilepsy well Network. 2018. Available at: https://managingepilepsywell.org/.
37. Pandey D. People living with epilepsy who live in high-crime neighborhoods experience significantly more seizures. New Orleans (LA): American Epilepsy Society; 2018.
38. Fantaneanu TA, Hurwitz S, van Meurs K, et al. Racial differences in Emergency Department visits for seizures. Seizure 2016;40:52–6.
39. Puka K, Smith ML, Moineddin R, et al. The influence of socioeconomic status on health resource utilization in pediatric epilepsy in a universal health insurance system. Epilepsia 2016;57(3):455–63.
40. Davoodvand S, Abbaszadeh A, Ahmadi F. Patient advocacy from the clinical nurses' viewpoint: a qualitative study. J Med Ethics Hist Med 2016;9:5.

Understanding Frontotemporal Disease Progression and Management Strategies

Malissa Mulkey, MSN, APRN, CCNS, CCRN, CNRN*

KEYWORDS

- Dementia • Cognitive deficits • Frontotemporal dementia • Early-onset dementia

KEY POINTS

- Dementia is defined as the loss of intellectual functions, including thinking, remembering, and reasoning, that is severe enough to interfere with an individual's daily functioning.
- Frontotemporal dementia (FTD) is a leading cause of early-onset dementia. FTD can present in the fourth and fifth decades and is associated with profound changes in behavior, personality, emotions, and cognition.
- Early detection and identification are needed to better support families' and caregivers' emotional and financial burdens. The purpose of this article is to increase FTD awareness and provide education to support clinicians.

Dementia is defined as the loss of intellectual functions, including thinking, remembering, and reasoning, severe enough to interfere with an individual's daily functioning. Frontotemporal dementia (FTD) is a leading cause of early-onset dementia. FTD can present in the fourth and fifth decades and is associated with profound changes in behavior, personality, emotions, and cognition. Early detection and identification are needed to better support families' and caregivers' emotional and financial burdens. The purpose of this article is to increase FTD awareness and provide education to support clinicians.

Dementia is a complex neurodegenerative chronic progressive syndrome. This mortal illness progresses over approximately 10 years from onset to death. It is a growing health problem affecting more than 5 million Americans.[1] Dementia leads to severe disability and a high burden for caregivers and costs to society. A systematic review described dementia as one of the strongest associated factors with nursing home admission.[2]

Advanced Clinical Practice, Duke University Hospital, 2301 Erwin RD, DUMC 3677, Durham, NC 27710, USA
* 35 Pearce Wood Court, Zebulon, NC 27597.
E-mail address: malissa.mulkey@duke.edu

Nurs Clin N Am 54 (2019) 437–448
https://doi.org/10.1016/j.cnur.2019.04.011
0029-6465/19/© 2019 Elsevier Inc. All rights reserved.
nursing.theclinics.com

Dementia is characterized by irreversible loss or decline in memory, cognition and other cognitive abilities, emotional control, social behavior, and motivation.[3,4] These changes result in reduced functional ability, a wide range of challenging behaviors, decreased ability to perform activities of daily living (ADLs), and a progressive need for support.[5] Transitions over time, however, are not uniform.[3]

FTD is a group of brain disorders or dementias that occur as a result of frontal and/or temporal lobe degeneration of the brain.[6] There is believed to be a strong genetic component to the disease, with a range of up to 40% heritability. Life expectancy for individuals with FTD is between 7 years and 13 years from symptom onset.[7] Although onset ranges from 21 years to 80 years, FTD typically occurs between ages 45 and 64. The younger onset often has a significantly greater effect on work, family, and economic burden compared with Alzheimer disease (AD).

The estimated prevalence of FTD in the United States is approximately 60,000 cases. FTD is the second most common cause of dementia for persons under the age of 65 and approximates that of early-onset AD.[8] FTD is significantly underrepresented because many providers are unfamiliar with this type of dementia. As a result, FTD frequently is misdiagnosed as AD, depression, Parkinson disease, or a psychiatric condition. Difficulty in identifying FTD often results in a 3-year to 4-year delay in obtaining accurate diagnosis and care.[8]

Some other names for FTD include frontotemporal lobar degeneration, frontal degeneration of non-Alzheimer type, presenile dementia, dementia of the frontal type, and Pick disease. FTD is different from other types of dementia in that memory usually is fairly well preserved, with gradual, progressive alterations in behavior, language, or movement.[9] Although memory seems preserved, on formal tests of episodic memory, patients with behavioral variant FTD (bvFTD) score in the same range as those with AD.[10] Other studies have found deficits in specific aspects of memory, such as personal autobiographical memory, future thinking, and imagination, with some of those deficiencies again as severe as those found in AD. Due to the similarities between FTD and autism spectrum disorder, researchers believe patients with FTD have an acquired deficit in cognitive capacity to attribute mental states to self and others.[8]

There are 2 clinical patterns of FTD: behavioral changes and language and communication difficulties.[8] bvFTD features a wide variety of behavioral impairments. Individuals with bvFTD have difficulty appreciating the mental state and perspective of others, contributing to an impairment in empathy, a source of considerable caregiver distress.[11] Studies evaluating emotional processing deficits and their relation to pathology of the orbitofrontal, anterior insular cortices, and amygdala regions in the brain have shown these areas are affected early in the course of bvFTD.[9,12] Alteration in sensitivity to social rewards also plays a role in the social cognitive deficits seen in bvFTD. In addition to alterations in emotion and insight, an individual with bvFTD often appears depressed, with lack of motivation or energy and personal hygiene neglect. Other behaviors include being easily distracted, repetitive/compulsive behaviors, exhibiting hypersexuality, and socially inappropriate behavior. Clinical studies focusing on apathy and disinhibition have identified these symptoms as causing the greatest caregiver distress. The bvFTD has been classified into apathetic (primary symptoms of aspontaneity, inertia, and slowness) and disinhibited (more distractibility, overactivity, and restlessness) behavioral presentations.[10]

Increased food consumption with a craving for sweet foods is a characteristic and discriminating feature of bvFTD. Subsequent studies investigated associations of this behavioral phenotype with metabolic and neuroanatomic characteristics.[13] This behavioral change is accompanied by alterations in cholesterol, insulin, neuroendocrine levels, and metabolic rate, having a significant effect on survival.

The second type of FTD presentation primarily centers around impairments in speech and language, such as expressive and receptive dysphasia, and may co-occur with the behavioral variant impairments.[13] Despite speech and language impairments, memory and spatial skills remain intact. Early work suggested that tests of spatial memory are helpful to discriminate between these 2 presentations. Changes in social cognition seen with the bvFTD also are found in the language presentations and in other FTD syndromes, including primary progressive aphasia, progressive supranuclear palsy, and corticobasal syndrome.

DISEASE PROGRESSION

The neuropathology of FTD is far more complex than that of AD.[8] Although not all FTD cases are familial, they usually are associated with a range of genetic mutations. There are 3 major patterns of disease progression, with wide variation in presentation and prognosis.[14] The first pattern presents with a tau protein inclusion pathology. The second pattern is TAR DNA-binding protein 43 (TDP-43) positive. The third pattern includes fused in sarcoma protein pathology. This third pattern is extremely rare, usually sporadic, with onset of symptoms at a younger age and frequently associated with neuropsychiatric symptoms. A significant number of individuals have an exceptionally long psychiatric prodrome whereas others deteriorate rapidly.[15] When baseline performance is equivalent, patients with bvFTD type have shown an annual rate of decline almost twice that of AD.[16] Although many FTD performance areas are similar to AD, some memory tasks decline twice as fast. This rapid decline in memory does not seem correlated with a faster spread of brain pathology.[8] Declines in memory and executive function are better explained by the degradation of the prefrontal cortices and their connections and are similar to the sequential pathologic changes seen in patients with bvFTD and TDP-43-positive pattern. Likewise, the comparatively slow decline in attention, orientation, and visuospatial tasks are related to posterior brain region sparing. It is believed that neurodegeneration is not diffuse or stochastic but follows a predictable and specific pattern. Using functional and structural magnetic resonance imaging, these patterns are determined primarily by involvement of large-scale networks critical to sensory, motor, and cognitive functions.[17] FTD predisposes an individual to physical complications, such as pneumonia, infection, and injury from a fall. The most common cause of death is pneumonia.[8]

Most individuals show clear evidence of decline over a 1-year to 3-year period, making this an important clinical diagnostic feature in the early clinical presentation.[18] The most common presentation of FTD has a mean survival from diagnosis of approximately 5 years and includes mood, personality, and behavioral changes that progress to frank dementia.[19] Although rare, some individuals have variants of FTD known as phenocopies that present with a slow decline or very slow progression. The presence of phenocopies further increases the difficulty of making an accurate diagnosis.[18]

Early Changes

Johannessen and colleagues[11] conducted a qualitative study with primary caregivers, usually spouses, to identify changes that occur as FTD progresses and their impact on the family. In the early stages of FTD the participants descriptions led to a theme called "sneaking signs" and was characterized by incomprehensive early signs and lack of insight. Participants described loved ones as having lack of insight and variations in normal personality, such as mood swings, tiredness, stress, and distraction.[9] During this time there often are signs of inability to absorb and remember information as well as a frequent and repeated need to ask for instructions. One area of particular challenge was driving because individuals were unable to determine the correct route even with well-known routes. Traffic citations for violations, such as driving too fast, commonly were reported. Individuals with FTD also tended to have significant early challenges with ADLs. These deficits have been correlated with increased impairments in executive functions, processing speeds, and more severe behavioral symptoms not associated with increased language impairment.[20] It is important to have comprehensive cognitive and behavioral evaluations at multiple time points to provide accurate and appropriate guidance and data to orient providers to an FTD diagnosis.[16] Because executive function has an impact on the ability to plan, organize, and sequence interventions, support in performing ADLs and other activities may be needed. Implementing strategies, such as placing items in appropriate sequential order and strategically posting reminders, initially may be helpful.[21]

Intermediate Phases

Because of significant impacts on the family, the intermediate phase often is the most disruptive and described as turning life upside down. In Johannessen and colleagues'[11] study, family members identified this phase as "the torment" due to the interference with work and vanishing social relations. Clinicians should prepare family for an increased risk of agitation and aggression, not just inhibition and apathy, any time a diagnosis of FTD is present or being ruled out. During this phase, individuals with FTD frequently exhibit a lack of initiative and passivity as they slowly become less able to perform daily activities on their own.[22] Working capacity declines with decreases in attention span and concentration. Some individuals experience interrupted sleep patterns, a lack of energy, and/or extreme restlessness. It is common for these individuals to develop a fear of being alone, to feel marked anxiety, and to develop feelings of helplessness that increase dependence on family.[11] As everyday routines and systems deteriorate, difficulties at work can result in an involuntary termination, leading to loss of meaningful occupation, social relations, and self-respect. Social networks shrink due to loss of social skills that offend others by coming off as rude, making social contact unpleasant. Over time, the individual and significant others are at high risk for becoming socially isolated. With appropriate support from a dementia specialist or psychologist, families can adapt to the diagnosis and the changes it brings and develop coping strategies. Family members and caregivers should be encouraged to share in the caregiving responsibilities to support family members living with an individual with FTD and prevent family breakdown.[23] Promoting a social network that includes relatives, friends, and support groups is important in mediating mood problems. Interventions targeting social participation may help reduce cognitive decline and mood problems.[24]

Relief with obtaining diagnosis

The pathway to a diagnosis often takes a long time.[11] The diagnostic work-up frequently is burdensome for patient and family, with multiple visits and tests. Unfortunately, general practitioners are not as knowledgeable about FTD, prolonging the process. In Johannessen and colleagues' work,[11] a diagnosis often was made during this intermediate phase and was described as a relief.

Later Stages

With disease progression, disabilities increase and the ability to communicate decreases, increasing dependence on others.[16] This is the beginning of the path to nursing home placement. Studies have shown patients with FTD are admitted to nursing homes significantly more often than patients with early-onset AD. This is believed to be due to the significant behavioral and personality changes that put a heavy strain on the caregivers.[9] Heavy strain can be from stress, depression; psychosocial, employment, and relationship problems; family conflict; financial difficulties; and quality of life.[25]

Dementia-specific training should be considered a way of potentially increasing care worker job satisfaction. Training has a significant positive impact on health care providers' confidence in understanding the experiences and social care needs of people with young-onset dementia and their families. This training improves practice by furthering their understanding of practical approaches to support patient care and empower people with young-onset dementia.[25]

When a patient and family resist nursing home placement, clinicians need to aid the family in the decision-making process.[11] Family should be encouraged to consider factors, including an individual's personality, stage, and interests. Additionally, the family must consider the increasing burden as the disease progresses. They should receive information on services and activities available at the nursing home. Family should obtain power of attorney before the patient reaches a point when the patient cannot give consent. If power of attorney is not obtained while the patient can consent, obtaining guardianship is required. Additionally, it is important to remember that the whole family is affected, including children and other family members.[11] Health systems should consider the increasing clinical and administrative burden of providing care as FTD progresses. These considerations include patient and family needs, increased time, and complexity of care coordination that must be allocated as a result of agitation/aggression, depression, dysphoria, anxiety, irritability, and lability.[26]

MEDICATIONS AND TREATMENT STRATEGIES

Medications that slow the disease progression of AD do not have the same effect for FTD.[14] Acetylcholinesterase inhibitors or N-methyl-D-aspartate receptor inhibitors provide no benefit for patients with FTD. Some studies have shown cognition is negatively impacted. Similarly, use of serotonin reuptake inhibitors have mixed results with treating challenging behaviors, such as agitation, aggression, and disinhibition. Implementation of behavioral strategies to address the lack of insight and awareness in bvFTD should be addressed and include changes associated with language variants.[8]

As with other dementias, care for individuals with FTD is provided predominantly by informal caregivers, including partners, family, and friends. There often are significant changes in an individual's ability to perform ADLs even at initial clinic presentation.[27] Significantly increased caregiver burden increases anxiety and stress and decreases a caregiver's sense of connection and overall psychological health and well-being. The effects on caregiver burden are associated with the patient's subtype and stage of dementia. The prevalence of higher levels of caregiver burden are increased greatly when an individual has bvFTD compared with other FTD subtypes or AD.[8] As disease progression occurs, behavioral changes increase that further compound the caregiver burden.

INTERVENTIONS AND BEHAVIORAL STRATEGIES

Reduced function in patients with FTD is associated most consistently with executive dysfunction and behavioral symptoms but is relatively independent of language deficits.[16] As a result, interventions that target the behavioral symptoms pathology are required regardless of clinical setting.[20] Interventions should be interdependent (between family or clinicians and the individual) rather than autonomous. Nurses often fail to provide sufficient reality orientation and validation therapy, a technique with proved efficacy,[28] nor do they regularly provide strategies that effectively have an impact on patient quality of life. Restraints are associated with increasing behavioral alterations, falls, and dependence as well as decreased cognitive function.[29] Multimodal interventions may provide better management of burdensome symptom and behavior, potentially improving functional outcomes and delaying transitions to costly long-term care.[20,26] Progressive muscle relaxation interventions have been shown to decrease anxiety, agitation, apathy, and irritability. Additionally, improvements in volition and social relationships often are realized (**Box 1**).[30]

COMMUNICATION

It is common for family caregivers to feel overwhelmed when developing effective communication strategies.[31] Communication can be difficult because of the cognitive impairments and decline in verbal skills. Sending and receiving information is impaired. The use of metaphors and combining humorous with literal statements may be particularly challenging to interpret. Although specific impairments may vary, they tend to center around word choice, building complex sentences, understanding verbal information, and remembering what was recently said.[32] The ability to send and receive nonverbal information or short easy sentences, however, and the ability to discuss things that happened a long time ago may remain intact. Because of challenges with verbal expression, patients exhibit nonverbal behavioral communication, such as agitation and aggression. High-quality research is limited; however, there are some theory-based strategies that may provide support, such as obtaining an individual's attention before attempting to communicate, speaking clearly, active-listening techniques, and making eye contact (see **Box 1**).[32]

BEHAVIORAL INTERVENTION STRATEGIES

Many individuals with FTD are not aware of their illness and, therefore, become frustrated with limitations or constraints. Separation from familiar environments and surroundings, such as during hospital admission, also increases anxiety.[33] Clinicians and family should be informed and alert for increased risk of agitation and aggression, not just inhibition and apathy, any time FTD is present or being ruled out. Increased anxiety may lead to agitation or other challenging behaviors, such as striking out at caregivers or resisting assistance. Aggressive behaviors may include shouting, name-calling, cursing, lewd comments, hitting, pushing, biting, pinching, scratching, grabbing, and disinhibited sexual behavior. When a patient's anxiety decreases, the challenging behaviors likely also decrease. Having management strategies and individualized approaches to ensure patient and staff safety and well-being requires understanding of the disease and careful planning. Effective management requires close collaboration between providers, staff, and families to develop and implement individualized care plans. Addressing staff concerns openly and supporting education about manifestations of FTD are important.

Anticipation and basic prevention strategies may reduce anxiety and agitation, thereby reducing a patient with FTD's need to exhibit challenging behaviors. Confrontation and correction usually are less successful than trying to prevent behaviors before they happen, thus reducing the risks involved if they do occur.[32,33] First and foremost, caregivers should remain calm. Smiling is useful because individuals with FTD understand positive emotional expressions better than negative ones.

Box 1
Prevention strategies to burdensome symptom and behavior

Communication
- Reduce overstimulation, including noise, people, or activity.
- Avoid confrontation. Do not argue or try to point out the truth.
- Do not make fun of an individual.
- Offer constant encouragement; maintain a calm voice.
- Acknowledge an individual's feelings.
- Use the same terms for care consistently, for example, in toileting.
- Using technology, such as iPads and software programs, can aid communication during early and intermediate phases.
- Make eye contact; use an even tone of voice and simplified language.
- Providing structure may help reduce inappropriate social behaviors.
- Ask individuals to remove their hand; then, gently remove their hand.
- Use a patient and calm approach and pleasant tone of voice. Responding with impatience or annoyance to a blank stare and lack of response to verbal requests could increase anxious or agitation.
- Singing—changing the words to familiar tunes or adding music may be helpful in gaining cooperation.

Assessment and observation
- Watch for signs agitation, such as pacing or yelling. Agitation often precedes aggression.
- Assess and treat pain or other illness.
- Evaluate benefits and side effects of medications closely and continuously.
- Track behavioral triggers and effective interventions.
- Report inappropriate touching immediately. A nurse should conduct a full body assessment immediately.

General strategies
- Use routine or rituals for easing daily care and promote cooperation
- Awareness of where an individual's hands are and prompt response help reduce inappropriate touching.
- Focus on positive interventions, discussion topics, and food to encourage compliance with regulations.
- Provide individualized activities that are success oriented. Group activities may be overwhelming.
- Provide information about a patient's "life story" for staff to facilitate conversation, socialization, and activity
- Encourage repetitive, safe, nondisruptive physical activities, such as folding wash clothes.

Managing roaming behaviors
- Include roaming in the daily routine.
- Routinely check feet for blisters.
- Avoid providing finger foods to avoid stopping for meals.
- Provide a box or bag of various items to rummage through.
- Walking beside persons and gradually slowing the pace may slow theirs.
- Using gentle prompts to encourage individuals to sit down may help them rest.
- Use soft music and soothing lighting during meals and sleep to reduce stimulation, promote relaxation, and decrease roaming.
- If routine roaming stops unexpectedly, assess for pain.

Approaches to personal care
- Break up tasks to reduce time.
- Assign same-gender staff to bathe.
- Modest staff apparel reduces visual triggers.
- Ensure privacy, go slowly, and explain each step before proceeding.
- Respect personal and intimate space. Allow an arm's-length distance when providing care.
- Provide something to hold or carry and/or a hands-on activity.
- A sitter, same-gender caregiver, and/or 2 staff members providing care may be necessary.

Compulsive behaviors
- Modify the environment and provide a replacement activity for unwanted behavior.
- Ignore nondangerous compulsive behaviors. Monitor and address nonsafe actions.

Disruptions to sleep and usual regimens may contribute to behavioral issues. It is important to maintain a routine when possible and, when necessary, make changes gradually.

Simple actions, such as using a patient's preferred name during conversations, can improve the therapeutic relationship, trust, and care.[34] Do not rush, argue, or touch an individual without permission and avoid startling a patient. Communication methods that strive to avoid arguments and escalate behavior, such as speaking in a soft pleasant voice, giving an individual enough room to respect personal space, and assigning consistent care providers, should be selected. Distraction and redirection to another activity are useful techniques to manage challenging behaviors with other types of dementia.[33] They usually are not effective, however, and worsen agitation in individuals with FTD, because cognitive abilities and memory often are retained. If possible, reduce the amount of stimulation to prevent escalation of negative behaviors (**Box 2**).

ADDRESSING CHALLENGING BEHAVIORS
Aggressive Behaviors

There may be physical aggression without warning, such as change in facial expression and body stance.[35] When behavior becomes aggressive, the best approach is to move away. It is important to intervene with confidence and respect. Calling for assistance may be needed if the individual becomes aggressive or risk to the patient or others escalates. To maintain safety, make sure there is an exit route and give the individual space (approximately 5 ft or 1.5 meters). Stand on the individual's least dominant side. Observe the location of the individual's arms and legs. Avoid attempts to reason or argue.[36] Validate the individual's emotions. Use a calm, slow, and lower voice to de-escalate agitation. Use single phrases and a directing voice to escort the person to a nearby area and engage in a positive activity.

Sexual Behaviors

Humans have an inherent capacity for sexual feelings. The way sexual feelings are displayed in public is based on social and cultural cues. Social guidelines define inappropriate actions and include those exhibited by a person living with FTD. Inappropriate actions may include increased or decreased sexual desire and disinhibited remarks and actions. When caregivers have a strong feeling of intimacy toward a patient, there often is the perception that the patient understands the caregiver's perspective or point of view. Disinhibition and hypersexuality can pose unique challenges in facility-based care centers. When dealing with inappropriate sexual behaviors,

---

Box 2
Address staff and caregiver concerns

- Provide education regarding behavior associated with the disease progression.
- Assist individuals with recognizing personality changes that may occur.
- Do not take a blank or threatening facial expression personally.
- Encourage sharing observations, concerns, and needs.
- Reinforce that the individual may not have normal reactions and feelings but there is no intent to hurt.
- Review possible triggers and implement positive approaches.

caregivers should not take the remarks or behavior personally. Using correction or punitive responses may be misinterpreted as abusive and result in agitation or aggression. Positive behavioral and environmental interventions are most effective. Responding with humor, distraction, and walking away often is effective. It is important for staff to report the behavior, determine the manifestations, and address the behavior quickly because delaying intervention results in worsening of the behavior.[35]

Working with caregivers to develop and individualize a home-based training program has had a positive impact on health-related quality of life.[37] Some areas of focus have included detecting and decreasing environmental stimuli to decrease agitation. It may be helpful to write a letter or work with storeowners if an individual has exhibited unacceptable behaviors, such as shoplifting, and have preemptive discussions with stores that are visited frequently. Having a prepared business-type card stating simply that the individual has an "Alzheimer-like disorder" to hand to individuals affected by inappropriate behavior that warrants an explanation may be helpful.[38] Encouraging caregivers to participate in social support groups has been found to assist with facing the increasing burden of providing care, decrease feelings of isolation, and provide helpful suggestions to assist with providing care and protect family caregivers.[39,40]

Roaming Behaviors

Individuals with FTD having a frequent need to be active can exhibit roaming behaviors. Roaming behaviors serve a purpose for the individual, such as reducing restlessness and stress, while also providing structure. Roaming should not be stopped entirely but may need to be adjusted and supervised. Roaming does not typically result in disorientation; however, safety and inappropriate behaviors, such as rudeness or appearing strange to other people, may be of concern. Safety measures are necessary to prevent injury while maintaining as much freedom as possible. Usually, individuals can navigate their surroundings, including returning to their starting point. These individuals typically go to the same place and follow the same route or pattern. If there are potential challenges along the path they are following, putting up a sign or blocking the route often redirects them to another route. Providing a safe protected area for roaming that is free of clutter and obstacles and nonskid footwear helps reduce injuries. Roaming and other physical activities burn calories and can lead to dehydration; therefore, monitoring intake and output is important.[35]

SUMMARY

FTD is the second most common form of dementia, typically occurring at an earlier age than other dementia types and having a steep decline, leading to an average life expectancy of between 7 years and 9 years.[8] The difference in presentation and younger age frequently lead to delayed diagnosis. As a result, a significant amount of patient, family, and caregiver stress occurs and may include financial impacts and negative effects on the family, including younger children.

Family and clinician caregivers frequently struggle with how to manage challenging behaviors. Despite the younger age, challenging behaviors exhibited by these individuals are more likely to require placement in long-term care.[41] When patients have difficulty with verbal communication, they often rely on behaviors to express themselves. When inappropriately managed, behaviors can escalate to physical aggression and injury. Because memory often is preserved until later in the disease process, strategies, such as distraction, are ineffective. Some themes for effective responses to undesired behaviors include avoiding conflict and implementing strategies that promote cooperation. FTD is challenging; therefore, the patient and family require support from a health care team. Implementing and teaching caregivers the proposed strategies presented in this article may help reduce frustrations everyone.

REFERENCES

1. American Psychiatric Association. Diagnostic and statistical manual of mentaldis-orders: DSM-5 2013. Available at: http://dsm.psychiatryonline.org/book.aspx?bookid5556. Accessed December 1, 2018.
2. Røen I, Selbæk G, Kirkevold Ø, et al. Resourse use and disease couse in dementia - nursing home (REDIC-NH), a longitudinal cohort study; design and patient characteristics at admission to Norwegian nursing homes. BMC Health Serv Res 2017;17:1–15.
3. Jutkowitz E, MacLehose RF, Gaugler JE, et al. Risk factors associated with cognitive, functional, and behavioral trajectories of newly diagnosed dementia patients. J Gerontol A Biol Sci Med Sci 2017;72(2):251–8.
4. Watanabe A, Suwa S. The mourning process of older people with dementia who lost their spouse. J Adv Nurs 2017;73(9):2143–55.
5. Prizer LP, Zimmerman S. Progressive support for activities of daily living for persons living with dementia. Gerontologist 2018;58:S74–87.
6. The Association for Frontotemporal Degeneration. Disease overview: what is FTD 2018. Available at: https://www.theaftd.org/what-is-ftd/disease-overview/. Accessed December 1, 2018.
7. Onyike CU, Diehl-Schmid J. The epidemiology of frontotemporal dementia. Int Rev Psychiatry 2013;25(2):130–7.
8. Hodges JR, Piguet O. Progress and challenges in frontotemporal dementia research: a 20-year review. J Alzheimers Dis 2018;62(3):1467–80.
9. Everhart DE, Watson EM, Bickel KL, et al. Right temporal lobe atrophy: a case that initially presented as excessive piety. Clin Neuropsychol 2015;29(7):1053–67.
10. O'Connor CM, Landin-Romero R, Clemson L, et al. Behavioral-variant frontotemporal dementia: distinct phenotypes with unique functional profiles. Neurology 2017;89(6):570–7.
11. Johannessen A, Helvik AS, Engedal K, et al. Experiences and needs of spouses of persons with young-onset frontotemporal lobe dementia during the progression of the disease. Scand J Caring Sci 2017;31(4):779–88.
12. Connor CM, Clemson L, Hornberger M, et al. Longitudinal change in everyday function and behavioral symptoms in frontotemporal dementia. Neurol Clin Pract 2016;6(5):419–28.
13. Poole ML, Brodtmann A, Darby D, et al. Motor speech phenotypes of frontotemporal dementia, primary progressive aphasia, and progressive apraxia of speech. J Speech Lang Hear Res 2017;60(4):897–911.
14. Shi L, Baird AL, Westwood S, et al. A decade of blood biomarkers for Alzheimer's disease research: an evolving field, improving study designs, and the challenge of replication. J Alzheimers Dis 2018;62(3):1181–98.
15. Gossink FT, Dols A, Kerssens CJ, et al. Psychiatric diagnoses underlying the phenocopy syndrome of behavioural variant frontotemporal dementia. J Neurol Neurosurg Psychiatry 2016;87(1):64–8.
16. Schubert S, Leyton CE, Hodges JR, et al. Longitudinal memory profiles in behavioral-variant frontotemporal dementia and Alzheimer's disease. J Alzheimers Dis 2016;51(3):775–82.

17. Filippi M, Agosta F, Ferraro PM. Charting frontotemporal dementia: from genes to networks. J Neuroimaging 2016;26(1):16–27.

18. Brodtmann A, Cowie T, McLean C, et al. Phenocopy or variant: a longitudinal study of very slowly progressive frontotemporal dementia. BMJ Case Rep 2013. https://doi.org/10.1136/bcr-2012-008077.

19. Lim D, Aradhye S. A case of fluctuating and stagnant frontotemporal dementia. J Am Geriatr Soc 2016;64(6):1380–1.

20. Moheb N, Mendez MF, Kremen SA, et al. Executive dysfunction and behavioral symptoms are associated with deficits in instrumental activities of daily living in frontotemporal dementia. Dement Geriatr Cogn Disord 2017;43(1/2):89–99.

21. Yu F, Vock DM, Barclay TR. Executive function: responses to aerobic exercise in Alzheimer's disease. Geriatr Nurs 2018;39(2):219–24.

22. Meijboom R, Steketee R, Koning I, et al. Functional connectivity and microstructural white matter changes in phenocopy frontotemporal dementia. Eur Radiol 2017;27(4):1352–60.

23. Hayo H. Diagnosis and support for younger people with dementia. Nurs Stand 2015;29(47):36–40.

24. Yates JA, Clare L, Woods RT. You've got a friend in me": can social networks mediate the relationship between mood and MCI? BMC Geriatr 2017;17:1–7.

25. Smith R, Ooms A, Greenwood N. Supporting people with young onset dementia and their families: an evaluation of a training course for care workers. Nurse Educ Pract 2017;27:7–12.

26. Sadak TI, Katon J, Beck C, et al. Key neuropsychiatric symptoms in common dementias: prevalence and implications for caregivers, clinicians, and health systems. Res Gerontol Nurs 2014;7(1):44–52.

27. Matsumoto N, Ikeda M, Fukuhara R, et al. Caregiver burden associated with behavioral and psychological symptoms of dementia in elderly people in the local community. Dement Geriatr Cogn Disord 2007;23(4):219–24.

28. Woods B, Aguirre E, Spector AE, et al. Cognitive stimulation to improve cognitive functioning in people with dementia. Cochrane Database Syst Rev 2012;(2):CD005562.

29. Sampaio FM, Sequeira C. Nurses' knowledge and practices in cases of acute and chronic confusion: a questionnaire survey. Perspect Psychiatr Care 2015; 51(2):98–105.

30. Ikemata S, Momose Y. Effects of a progressive muscle relaxation intervention on dementia symptoms, activities of daily living, and immune function in group home residents with dementia in Japan. Jpn J Nurs Sci 2017;14(2):135–45.

31. Hayajneh FA, Shehadeh A. The impact of adopting person-centred care approach for people with Alzheimer's on professional caregivers' burden: an interventional study. Int J Nurs Pract 2014;20(4):438–45.

32. Machiels M, Metzelthin SF, Hamers JPH, et al. Interventions to improve communication between people with dementia and nursing staff during daily nursing care: a systematic review. Int J Nurs Stud 2017;66:37–46.

33. Pfeifer P, Vandenhouten C, Purvis S, et al. The impact of education on certified nursing assistants' identification of strategies to manage behaviors associated with dementia. J Nurses Prof Dev 2018;34(1):26–30.

34. Moore A. Compassionate care. Nurs Stand 2014;28(28):61.

35. Davison TE, McCabe MP, Bird M, et al. Behavioral symptoms of dementia that present management difficulties in nursing homes: staff perceptions and their concordance with informant scales. J Gerontol Nurs 2017;43(1):34–43.

36. Graham F. A new frontier: improving nursing care for people with dementia and delirium in hospitals. J Nurs Adm 2015;45(12):589–91.
37. Kuo L-M, Huang H-L, Liang J, et al. Trajectories of health-related quality of life among family caregivers of individuals with dementia: a home-based caregiver-training program matters. Geriatr Nurs 2017;38(2):124–32.
38. Merrilees J, Hubbard E, Mastick J, et al. Sleep in persons with frontotemporal dementia and their family caregivers. Nurs Res 2014;63(2):129–36.
39. Kucukguclu O, Akpinar Soylemez B, Yener G, et al. The effects of support groups on dementia caregivers: a mixed method study. Geriatr Nurs 2018;39(2):151–6.
40. Yang CT, Liu HY, Shyu YI. Dyadic relational resources and role strain in family caregivers of persons living with dementia at home: a cross-sectional survey. Int J Nurs Stud 2014;51(4):593–602.
41. Hvidsten L, Engedal K, Selbaek G, et al. Quality of life in people with young-onset alzheimer's dementia and frontotemporal dementia. Dement Geriatr Cogn Disord 2018;45(1–2):91–104.

An International Perspective of Transition of Neurological Disease
The Latin American and the Caribbean Region

Stefany Ortega-Perez, RN, MSc, PhD(c)[a],[*],
Lorena Sanchez-Rubio, RN, MSN, PhD(c)[b],
Roxana De las Salas, RN, MSc, PhD(c)[a],
Juana Borja-Gonzalez, RN, MSN, PhD(c)[a]

KEYWORDS

- Latin America • Neurologic disorders • Health transition • Neuroscience nursing
- Nursing care

KEY POINTS

- In Latin America and the Caribbean (LAC) region, a significant proportion of risk factors can be attributed to classic preventable cardiovascular diseases.
- There are important differences in demographics, socioeconomic status and injury mechanisms that may influence the patient's outcome.
- Current treatments are variable and depend on causes, prognosis, symptoms, sequelae, and complications.
- After disease progression, the greatest burden of disease will likely fall on the caregiver.
- The practice of neuroscience nursing is taking a turn to inquire about the needs of the patient and family during the long transition to home.

THE LATIN AMERICA AND THE CARIBBEAN REGION

The Latin America and the Caribbean (LAC) region consists of 33 countries, roughly 600 million people, with a large proportion are of low-income and middle-income countries (LMICs). Approximately 36% of the region's population is living at or below the poverty line.[1,2] Based on this, neurologic injury disorders disproportionately affect

Disclosure Statement: The authors state that they have no conflict of interest.
[a] Nursing Department, Universidad del Norte, Km 5 via a Puerto Colombia, Área Metropolitana de Barranquilla, Barranquilla, Colombia; [b] Nursing Department, Universidad del Tolima, Calle 42 #1b-1, Ibagué, Colombia, Colciencias 727
* Corresponding author. Universidad del Norte, Km 5 via a Puerto Colombia, Área Metropolitana de Barranquilla, Barranquilla, Colombia, Colciencias 757.
E-mail address: srortega@uninorte.edu.co

this population, which faces not only most risk factors, but also has less developed health systems to manage patient health outcomes.[2]

The Epidemiologic Transition

Demographic characteristics have changed significantly in the LAC region over the past 25 years, the population growth and aging of the population is catching up with that of high-income countries (HICs). Expectedly, the burden of disease has also evolved. Alzheimer disease (AD), traumatic brain injury (TBI), and stroke are now in the most common causes of disability-adjusted life-years, years of life lost, and years lived with disability.[3] These changes have forced health systems, which had traditionally been dedicated to the care of acute neurologic diseases, to focus their attention on the complex and multidisciplinary needs of people with chronic neurologic diseases, yet this system needs continued improvement.

The Risk Factors

The pathophysiology of neurologic diseases is likely similar worldwide. In the LAC region, a significant proportion of the risk factors can be attributed to classic preventable cardiovascular factors, such as hypertension, diabetes, and smoking, although there are important differences in demographics, socioeconomic status, and injury mechanisms that may influence the patient's outcome: patients are younger, delay arrival to the hospital, and are more likely to have been involved in a motorcycle or pedestrian road traffic accident.[4,5] The region has reported the highest incidence rate of intracranial injury worldwide, because of high rates of road traffic crashes and violence.[5]

The impact of long-term neurologic disability is greatest in LAC because of several conditions that increase the risk and contribute to injury and premature death. The high use of motorcycles: without helmets, while speeding, while drunk driving, lacking seat belts, and with inadequate protection for children only increases the risk of injury.[6,7] The vector-borne diseases such as Zika and Chagas are a major public health problem in the region. These diseases may result in serious neurologic complications: destruction of the nervous system (Chagas), Guillain-Barré syndrome, and microcephaly (Zika).[8] There is no vaccine for either disease; vector control is the most effective method of protecting population from infection. The objective of vector control is to reduce the mosquito population, and avoid breeding sites and the vector's contact with humans.[9] Finally, socioeconomic status can heighten the risk through several mechanisms: limited access to health care, unhealthy lifestyles, poor knowledge and compliance with prevention strategies, increased stress, and underdiagnosis of severe cardiovascular diseases.

Prehospital Emergency Care

Prehospital care is an important aspect in the management of the acute neurologic patient. This care should be delivered by trained personnel in an organized emergency medical services system to reduce mortality and improve outcomes. In general, prehospital care capabilities in LMICs are less developed especially in rural areas, where utilization of formal emergency medical services was often very low. The variation in the transport to the hospital includes commercial and taxi drivers, volunteers, and other bystanders who provide a large proportion of prehospital transport, and occasionally first aid.[10] In many LMICs, transport in an ambulance does not ensure access to resuscitation. "The services provided by prehospital emergency transport vehicles can vary from life support provided by physicians to 'scoop and run' assistance provided by minimally trained technicians."[1] Prehospital care, without resuscitation, may result in secondary brain injury that worsens the severity and contributes to poor outcomes. Bonow and colleagues[5] state "patients who were healthy enough to survive the long transport survived, whereas those who were more severely injured may have died of their injuries before reaching the hospital." However, studies in this field cannot draw conclusions about the influence of prehospital care and patients outcomes. These studies provide valuable information that will strengthen prehospital care in the LAC region.[1,5]

Acute Treatment

It is well-known that primary prevention has an important role in the control of neurologic diseases around the world, especially in LMICs. Secondary brain injury (SBI) is a major cause of poor neurologic outcomes. However, aspects of acute care and SBI prevention are still largely neglected in these countries.[11] Patients with neurologic disease are stabilized on arrival to the emergency department, but a bed in the intensive care unit (ICU) may not be immediately available. In spite of this situation, the ICUs meet the requirements to care for high-complexity patients, based mostly in a traditional imaging and clinical examination.

The management of patients in most countries in the LAC region is based on imaging and clinical examination (ICE); although international guidelines provide a basis for neuromonitoring of intracranial pressure (ICP) to assess and manage intracranial hypertension. It is evident that most neurocritical patients are being managed without ICP monitoring in the LAC. Procedures are lacking in Latin America on which method has the best impact on patients; hence, it is critical to develop management, treatment, and care guidelines based on the special conditions of the region.[6]

The most relevant literature about neuromonitoring protocols for the LAC region are based on the BEST TRIP trial (Benchmark Evidence from South American Trials: Treatment of Intracranial Pressure).[12] The objective of this trial was to compare outcomes between patients with severe TBI managed using ICP monitoring (ICP group) and those managed using a protocol in which treatment was based on the ICE group in ICUs in Bolivia and Ecuador. The results showed no significant between-group differences in primary outcomes (reduced mortality and improved neuropsychological and functional recovery at 6 months), although there was a trend toward lower mortality and more efficient care in the ICP group. BEST TRIP supported that management guidelines are needed for places in which ICP monitoring is not the standard of care, and the development of consensus-based protocol for severe TBI treatment without ICP monitoring.

Care Transition from Hospital to Home

Although the ICU-level care received by all patients is similar to the international guidelines, the interventions received after the patient leaves the ICU depend heavily on family resources.[5] For the neurologic patient, early discharge from hospital to home has become a strategy to reduce hospital stay and complications.[13] Discharge planning often includes patient education, promotion of self-management, and outpatient follow-up. Of patients who survived to hospital discharge, few are discharged to a formal care setting, to a rehabilitation facility, or have a discharge plan.[1] The out-of-pocket cost for these services are excessive for many families and the cost can become a burden, thus limiting the option of postinjury rehabilitation.[5]

Hospital managers and care providers in the LAC need to implement discharge strategies to prevent adverse events, emergency department return visits, and hospital readmissions within 30 days of discharge. However, the information available on effective discharge strategies for patients and their families in the LAC region is limited. This continues to be an approach that is not commonly used, particularly in relation to hospital-to-home discharge planning, with fragmentation in postdischarge care.[14] Nurses play a leading role in this care transition. The international literature about care transition, carried out by nurses, from hospital to home has increased in the past 5 years, mainly in HICs from North America, Europe, and Asia. Although there is growing importance of this topic, there is a lack of research in this area in the LAC region.[14]

Carer's Transitions

Individuals with neurologic disorders experience physical, cognitive, and emotional problems that disturb their capability to live independently and frequently need permanent assistance for their everyday life activities. In most LAC region countries, this assistance is mainly provided by family members, who become the primary carer. However, the carer's transition has not been taken into account; discharge care plans are often formulated and delivered very close to patient discharge from the hospital, which can lead to a buildup of information, future uncertainties, and lack of care safety.[14] Hence, it is necessary to provide services for carers (eg, guidance and practical assistance) and it is imperative to develop and implement health care strategies to meet the needs of the carers.[15]

REGION-SPECIFIC NEUROLOGIC DISEASES

Neurologic disorders in the LAC region are among the main sources of disability.[16,17] The burden of neurologic disease in the LAC region is associated with stroke, neurodegenerative disorders, and also the consequences of the Zika virus in 2013.[18] With this range of disorders, current treatments are variable and depend on their causes, prognosis, symptoms, sequelae, and future complications.

Microcephaly by Zika Virus

The microcephaly product of the Zika virus is a life-long condition and has no cure or treatment. Children with microcephaly will need treatment for seizure management; developmental delay; intellectual disability; and problems with movement, balance, feeding, swallowing, and hearing and vision loss. Early intervention may include speech, occupational, and physical therapies.[19,20] Many nurses hold lead positions in health education, health promotion, and health surveillance to identify, prevent, and manage Zika virus. Strategies may involve going door-to-door to educate individuals and entire communities about preventing transmission and protecting themselves from the disease.[21]

Use of Medical Marijuana

Thanks to the development of clinical research in United States and Europe and the legalization of medical marijuana,[22,23] some countries in the LAC region (Chile, Puerto Rico, Uruguay, and Colombia) have contemplated using medical marijuana as a treatment for diseases such as epilepsy. Preliminary data from human studies suggest that cannabis, especially cannabidiol, is effective in the treatment of some patients with epilepsy. However, the data available for the LAC region are limited and do not show definitive conclusions. Only randomized clinical trials will provide comprehensive information on the efficacy and safety of use. To perform these trials, it is necessary to have legislation authorizing the use of cannabis for neurologic diseases.[24]

Stroke

The epidemiologic transition to aging in the LAC region has led to an increase in cardiovascular risk factors such as hypertension, smoking, abdominal obesity, poor eating habits, sedentary lifestyle, diabetes, alcoholism, and dyslipidemias. All of these factors have an impact on morbidity and mortality from stroke. Stroke is the leading cause of death in most LACs and is considered preventable. Patients who survive a stroke quite often have marked physical and functional disability, necessitating rehabilitation.[17] Worldwide stroke prevention has focused on reducing blood pressure or cholesterol using pharmacologic and lifestyle interventions. Several countries in the LAC region have implemented national noncommunicable diseases programs and have taken policy measures to reduce tobacco and alcohol use, increase physical activities, and encourage healthy dietary practices.[25] For acute care, the ischemic stroke guidelines recommend intravenous thrombolytic therapy with recombinant tissue plasminogen activator (rt-PA).[26,27] The experience of a hospital in the Colombian Caribbean has shown this strategy to reduce disability levels in patients when the medication and a multidisciplinary team trained to minimize delays is used ensure the possibility of greater success.[28]

Neurocognitive Disorders

A multicenter study conducted in Brazil, Cuba, Chile, Peru, and Venezuela showed that the global prevalence of dementia in Latin America is 7.1% (95% confidence interval 6.8–7.4) with AD being the most frequent type. Cholinesterase inhibitors (galantamine, rivastigmine, donepezil) are prescribed for the treatment of mild to moderate-grade symptoms of AD; however, they may lose effectiveness after 12 weeks of starting treatment and are not indicated in more advanced stages ($\geq$6 score on global deterioration scale and Functional Analysis Screening Tool scale phase $\geq$6).[29] Memantine, another of the drugs used, is a noncompetitive N-methyl-D-aspartate receptor antagonist. Cholinesterase inhibitors and/or memantine help decrease symptoms, but do not slow the course of disease.[30] They are combined with other medications to control symptoms such as depression, agitation, sleep disturbances, or subsequent complications such as sphincter incontinence, urinary tract infections, pressure ulcers, and thrombophlebitis caused by immobility. In addition, adverse effects such as diarrhea, dizziness, loss of appetite, cramps, nausea, fatigue, insomnia, vomiting, weight loss, and hepatotoxicity can occur.[31] This indicates that after disease progression, the greatest burden of disease will fall on the carer.

In Parkinson disease, drug treatments have focused on increasing dopamine levels (dopamine agonists, catechol-O-methyltransferase inhibitors, monoamine oxidase type B enzyme inhibitors), and decreasing symptoms associated with gait problems, movement, and tremor reduction (anticholinergics).[32] A Cuban study found a possible neuroprotective effect of human erythropoietin but suggests further research.[33] Procedures such as physiotherapy, occupational and speech therapy, cognitive training, and deep brain stimulation, as well as noninvasive brain stimulation strategies have been indicated in the LAC region.[34] However, receiving this treatment depends on the patient or family's ability to afford treatment.

NEUROSCIENCE NURSING EDUCATION IN THE LATIN AMERICA AND THE CARIBBEAN REGION

In the LAC region, many people cannot access complete health services to achieve a healthy life, prevent disease, or receive primary health care in a timely manner.[35] The number of nursing professionals in the region is scarce, related to the needs of the populations and is concentrated in the capitals; therefore, access to health services in peripheral areas is difficult. In terms of human resources for nursing, there is a wide variation both among the countries of the LAC region and within each of them. The proportion of nurses (registered nurses and certified nursing assistants) per 10,000 inhabitants ranges from 81.3 in Cuba to 3.5 in Haiti. The median is 10.4 nurses per 10,000 inhabitants.[36]

Nurses are vital members of the health care team. Therefore, it is essential to ensure that nursing education prepares students to respond to the needs of health systems and to work collaboratively with the health care team.[37] In the LAC region, nurses are prepared in specializations that enrich their knowledge of the care of critically ill patients. These specialists or advanced practice nurses strengthen the clinical fields; however, there is little clarity regarding the legislation and their recognition by the health system and the institutions in which they work. This makes it difficult for nurses to access higher levels of education. Therefore, it is necessary to increase and improve training programs.[38]

In the LAC region, there are 246 schools of nursing, and 51 doctoral programs in nursing, with the greatest concentration in Brazil (37 programs).[35] Nurses who provide care in ICUs are a fundamental part of the management and recovery of neurocritical patients, and their work is based on management guides adapted in the medical model. Although the curricula of the nursing schools in the region comply with the guidelines of the American Association of Nursing College[39] regarding the topics considered essential in teaching, the topics related to follow-up, management of complications, rehabilitation processes that are relevant when talking about the transition of the neurocritical patients, and that are related to the evaluation and continuous improvement of health programs, continue to be scarce. Despite the existence of public policies, the issue of disability has not reached the visibility required because of deficient implementation of knowledge among officials and public entities, making it difficult to coordinate nursing care with the health care team, and a persistent disconnection in the continuity of care.

In recent years, the focus of the scientific community has been on grouping efforts to analyze the characteristics of neurologic care in Latin America and create care guidelines that are applicable under the conditions of this region.[40] Some efforts have been made, like the BEST TRIP trial,[41] but it is urgent and necessary to continue working on this.

SUMMARY

The transitions of neurologic diseases in the LAC region are impacted by specific factors to this region (eg, Zika and Chagas). Important barriers exist, including limited access to prehospital emergency care, lack of equipment and neuromonitoring, and availability of services at reasonable distance and cost to patients and their families. Despite these needs, nurses are working hard every day to achieve favorable patient outcomes. It is a priority to develop care guidelines based on the specific conditions of the LAC region.

REFERENCES

1. Celix JM. Severe traumatic brain injury in South America: the association between resources and outcomes. [ProQuest Diss Theses] Repository 2013.

2. Puvanachandra P, Hyder AA. Traumatic brain injury in Latin America and the Caribbean: a call for research. Salud Publica Mex 2008;50(Suppl 1):S3–5.

3. Lancet Neurology. A neurology revival in Latin America. Lancet Neurol 2015; 14(12):1143.
4. Neurological Disorders Collaborator Group. Global, regional, and national burden of neurological disorders during 1990–2015: a systematic analysis for the Global Burden of Disease Study 2015. Lancet Neurol 2017;16:877–97.
5. Bonow RH, Barber J, Temkin NR, et al. The outcome of severe traumatic brain injury in Latin America. World Neurosurg 2018;111:2–5.
6. Hendrickson P, Pridgeon J, Temkin NR, et al. Development of a severe traumatic brain injury consensus-based treatment protocol conference in Latin America. World Neurosurg 2018;110:e952–7.
7. Johnson WD, Griswold DP. Traumatic brain injury: a global challenge. Lancet Neurol 2017;16(12):949–50.
8. Amela Heras C, José M, Moros S. Vector-transmitted diseases. A new challenge for public health surveillance systems. Gac Sanit 2016;30(3):167–9.
9. PAHO, WHO. Integrated vector management: a comprehensive response to vector-borne diseases. 48th Directing Council. 60th Session of the Regional Committee 2008. Available at: http://www1.paho.org/english/GOV/CD/cd48-13-e.pdf?ua=1. Accessed December 20, 2018.
10. Nielsen K, Mock C, Joshipura M, et al. Assessment of the status of prehospital care in 13 low- and middle-income countries. Prehosp Emerg Care 2012;16(3): 381–9.
11. Ortega-Pérez S, Amaya-Rey MC. Secondary brain injury: a concept analysis. J Neurosci Nurs 2018;54(4):220–4.
12. Chesnut RM, Temkin N, Carney N, et al. A trial of intracranial-pressure monitoring in traumatic brain injury. N Engl J Med 2012;367(26):2471–81.
13. Rivera D, Perrin PB, Senra H, et al. Development of the family needs assessment tool for caregivers of individuals with neurological conditions in Latin America. Psicol desde el Caribe 2013;30(1):1–20.
14. Lima M, Magalhães A, Oelke N, et al. Care transition strategies in Latin American countries: an integrative review. Rev Gaucha Enferm 2018;39:1–11.
15. Manes F. The huge burden of dementia in Latin America. Lancet Neurol 2016; 15(1):29.
16. Negrotto L, Correale J. Evolution of multiple sclerosis prevalence and phenotype in Latin America. Mult Scler Relat Disord 2018;22:97–102.
17. Avezum Á, Costa-Filho FF, Pieri A, et al. Stroke in Latin America: burden of disease and opportunities for prevention. Glob Heart 2015;10(4):323–31.
18. Bonilla-Soto L. Zika virus in the Americas: an environmental health. P R Health Sci J 2018;37(Special issue):S5–14.
19. Hurtado-Villa P, Puerto A, Victoria S, et al. Raised frequency of microcephaly related to zika virus infection in two birth defects surveillance systems in Bogotá and Cali, Colombia. Pediatr Infect Dis J 2017;36(10):1017–9.
20. Magalhaes-Barbosa M, Prata-Barbosa A, Robaina J, et al. Trends of the microcephaly and Zika virus outbreak in Brazil, January-July 2016. Travel Med Infect Dis 2016;14(5):458–63.
21. Wilson A, Nguyen TN. The zika virus epidemic: public health roles for nurses. Online J Issues Nurs 2017;22(1):1–9.
22. Devinsky O, Marsh E, Friedman D, et al. Cannabidiol in patients with treatment-resistant epilepsy: an open-label interventional trial. Lancet Neurol 2016;15(3): 270–8.
23. Friedman D, Devinsky O. Cannabinoids in the treatment of epilepsy. N Engl J Med 2015;373(11):1048–58.

24. Kochen S. Cannabis use in epilepsy. Current situation in Argentina and abroad. Vertex 2016;XXVII(130):457–62.
25. Kalkonde YV, Alladi S, Kaul S, et al. Stroke prevention strategies in the developing world. Stroke 2018;49:3092–7.
26. Lees KR, Bluhmki E, von Kummer R, et al. Time to treatment with intravenous alteplase and outcome in stroke: an updated pooled analysis of ECASS, ATLANTIS, NINDS, and EPITHET trials. Lancet 2010;375(9727):1695–703.
27. Sila C. Finding the right t-PA dose for Asians with acute ischemic stroke. N Engl J Med 2016;374(24):2389–90.
28. Hernández E, Guarín E, Lora F, et al. Trombólisis intravenosa en pacientes con accidente cerebrovascular isquémico: Experiencia de un Hospital del Caribe Colombiano. Acta Neurol Colomb 2017;33(1):3–7.
29. Custodio N, Wheelock A, Thumala D, et al. Dementia in Latin America: epidemiological evidence and implications for public policy. Front Aging Neurosci 2017; 9(JUL):1–11.
30. Prescrire Rédaction. Pour mieux soigner, des médicaments à écarter: bilan 2018. Rev Prescrire 2018;38(412):135–44.
31. Cardona-Gómez G, Lopera F. Dementia, preclinical studies in neurodegeneration and its potential for translational medicine in South America. Front Aging Neurosci 2016;8:304.
32. Marin D, Carmona H, Ibarra M, et al. Enfermedad de Parkinson: fisiopatología, diagnóstico y tratamiento. Rev Univ Ind Santander Salud 2018;50(1):79–92.
33. Pedroso I, Bringas M, Aguiar A, et al. Use of Cuban recombinant human erythropoietin in Parkinson's disease treatment. MEDICC Rev 2012;14(1):11–7.
34. Witt K, Kalbe E, Erasmi R, et al. Nonpharmacological treatment procedures for Parkinson's disease. Nervenarzt 2017;88(4):383–90.
35. Cassiani S, Wilson L, Mikael S, et al. The situation of nursing education in Latin America and the Caribbean towards universal health. Rev Lat Am Enfermagem 2017;25:e2913.
36. Pan American Health Organization. Ampliación del rol de las enfermeras y enfermeros en la atención primaria de salud 2018. Available at: http://iris.paho.org/xmlui/handle/123456789/34959. Accessed December 20, 2018.
37. World Health Organization. Global standards for the initial education of professional nurses and midwives. Geneva (Switzerland): WHO; 2009.
38. Punchak M, Mukhopadhyay S, Sachdev S, et al. Neurosurgical care: availability and access in low-income and middle-income countries. World Neurosurg 2018; 112:e240–54.
39. Zug KE, Cassiani SH, Pulcini J, et al. Advanced practice nursing in Latin America and the Caribbean: regulation, education and practice. Rev Lat Am Enfermagem 2016;24(0):e2807.
40. Mejia-Mantilla JH, Aristizabal-Mayor JD. Capacidad operativa de las unidades de cuidados intensivos colombianas y latinoamericanas en el manejo de la hemorragia subaracnoidea: un acercamiento preliminar. Acta Colomb Cuid Intensivo 2017;17(4):241–6.
41. Chesnut R, Bleck T, Citerio G, et al. A consensus-based interpretation of the BEST TRIP ICP trial. J Neurotrauma 2015;32(22):1722–4.

CPI Antony Rowe
Eastbourne, UK
July 29, 2019